This book belongs to:

BALANCE

is

BULLSH*T

BALANCE IS

Bullsh*t

A REALISTIC APPROACH TO INTEGRATING
HEALTHIER HABITS INTO YOUR LIFE

ALICIA McKENZIE

ILLUSTRATIONS BY
REGINA SHKLOVSKY

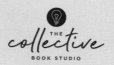

THE
collective
BOOK STUDIO

physical wellness

community wellness

mental wellness

financial wellness

FOREWORD

I have had the good fortune of knowing and working with Alicia for several years now. Watching her juggle everything that life has to offer is simply remarkable. Whether it is fitness, family (five kids!), business, or serving her community, she is an example that we can all model ourselves after. To say that she is someone that I greatly respect and admire is an understatement. I was quite humbled when she asked me to write the foreword for her book.

As you'll discover in *Balance Is Bullsh*t*, handling all of life's duties requires having good habits and systems in place. We all have a ton of things going on in life, and it's far too easy to use the excuse that we're too busy. Our minds like to automate to conserve as much energy as possible, and this is where habits come in. It seems that much of our life is automated and we're running on autopilot. This can be a good thing or a bad thing depending on the habits that we've developed. If we can create good, healthy habits, being on autopilot is fantastic. On the flip side, heading into a crash landing on autopilot because of our unhealthy habits is not what we're aiming for.

It's important to recognize that creating healthy habits is not an easy process. It may sound simple to just stop scrolling social media and instead shift some of that time toward yourself, but it's certainly not easy when we're used to doing it for hours a day for multiple years! If you know this ahead of time, it can help ease the transition to making conscious choices to change your daily habits. Don't expect to suddenly be the epitome of health and wellness on day one; accept that it's perfectly okay for it to be a process!

In my personal life, there are several habits that I aim for daily. I will also be the first to admit that I'm far from perfect and I'm always trying to improve myself. There are days when everything on my list doesn't get done, but I don't beat myself up too much about it. There's a lesson to be learned in the power of consistency over the long term. If we can harness the power of incremental progress, we're much more likely to be better off in the long run.

For my daily habits, I always aim for a few basics every single day. I aim to train with weights at least four times a week. I aim to do some form of cardio every single day, even if that's just taking a short walk in the neighborhood. I try to get in at least ten minutes of mindfulness practice daily so that I am more self-aware and in better control of my emotions. I also love reading and have created the habit of reading each day. I also make it a point to help do the dishes every morning, whether that's unloading the dishwasher or washing some by hand. I've also found that listening to a podcast or an audio-book makes doing the dishes a lot easier, and I usually end up in the good graces of my wife for helping her out! I have a few more daily habits, but those are the basics.

These habits are not something I've always done. As I've gotten older and wiser, they are practices that I have developed for my long-term wellbeing and self-improvement. With the year that was 2020, I chose to embed these habits into my lifestyle; otherwise it would have been far too easy to dwell on all the negativity in the world. I chose to make some good come from being stuck at home. I knew that if I was going to be home, I had the opportunity to really keep to these habits without the demands of travel. Something important to remember is that no matter what happens to us, we always have the ability to control our response to it. No matter how bad things might seem, chances are we can find some good to come from it. In 2020, my young and healthy wife was diagnosed with breast cancer, had multiple surgeries, was in the hospital for days at a time, and underwent chemotherapy. Meanwhile, like most families, we were homeschooling two young kids and dealing with the reality of COVID-19 and a very serious quarantine. Despite all this, I feel that we came out of the year better than ever. We owe it a lot to the daily habits that we implemented and the positive mindset that we kept through it all. Life is tough at times, but chances are we can take away some key lessons from the worst of times and ultimately come out better in the long run.

As you'll read in this book, it's also important to build good habits beyond fitness and mental health. If you extend these good habits into other areas of your life, such as personal finances and strengthening your community, you will greatly enhance the amount of good you can do in the world. One of my favorite financial rules that crosses over perfectly from fitness is focusing on delayed gratification. While it might sound appealing to sit around binge-watching Netflix and eating popcorn every night, if we do it at the expense of our fitness regimen, it will be detrimental in the long run. The same holds true for our personal finances. If we aim to impress others with fancy purchases, it may feel good to show it off in that moment, but it may not be the best use of our finances in the long term. It's absolutely imperative to make sure that you are paying yourself first and always saving for the future. By having a long-term time horizon for both finance and fitness, you are headed for a better life down the road. And like Alicia and her husband, I certainly aspire to teach my kids the importance of financial literacy using fun exercises.

Similarly, serving our community has several benefits. We're helping others, of course, but it's also important to know that in doing so we're also helping ourselves. There's no greater feeling in the world then being able to give and make a difference in the lives of others. I've experienced this firsthand through Renaissance Periodization, helping hundreds of thousands of folks change their lives for the better through proper nutrition and fitness. Watching Alicia and her family serve their community has been a big inspiration for me, and I encourage everyone to get out there and help yourself by helping others in whatever ways you can.

Alicia is someone that I am honored to have gotten to know over the past few years. I know you're in the best of hands with her. Using the principles laid out in this book will no doubt have a big impact on your life. Best of luck on your journey to building healthy habits that last a lifetime!

—Nick Shaw, CEO and Founder of
Renaissance Periodization

INTRODUCTION

For me, life is about keeping balls in the air. As a former USA weightlifting and CrossFit athlete, I have over a decade of experience in the fitness industry, a multitude of certifications including but not limited to nutrition, personal training, gymnastics, and mobility, and have done everything from competing at a high level to owning and operating a gym for five years. I have coached many amazing people and provided them the tools to accomplish their wellness goals. I am fortunate enough to have lived and breathed every facet of the health and wellness industry, and I started a family while doing it. I've won weightlifting competitions while breastfeeding and pumping behind the scenes.

Often, it feels like I'm juggling ten balls at the same time. Most of them are rubber, but several—physical, mental, community, and financial wellness—are glass. It's okay if I drop any of the rubber balls, because when they hit the ground they'll bounce and I'll adjust to keep the others in the air. But if I drop any of the glass balls, they won't bounce, they'll break, and that's when I'm going to have issues! Does this mean that I don't ever drop balls? Of course not. It just means that I'm good at discerning which balls will bounce and which won't. I'm here to help you do the same.

As a wife, an entrepreneur, and the mother of a small basketball team, I've learned a thing or two about juggling. I have experienced challenges and obstacles in every part of my life, but with a little hard work, a lot of intention, and the help of my village, I have been able to achieve some amazing things. Through trial and error, I implemented a plan, and over the years this plan has evolved into a sustainable lifestyle and program. Now I'd like to share it with you.

BALANCE IS BULLSH*T

We've all heard the phrase "work/life balance." I want to get this out of the way: Balance is bullshit. The mere definition of balance is so wrong when used in the context of our lives.

 balance: *a condition in which different elements are equal or in the correct proportions*

Life can be unpredictable and messy. And for that reason, I'd like to provide you with a different narrative. I don't think the elements of my life have ever been balanced in equal proportions, and that's okay. I have learned that it is possible to seamlessly integrate all the facets of my life by coming to grips with the fact that everything evolves and changes, with or without my control.

The key is to focus on the four aspects of life that mean the most, the things we can control:

Physical Wellness, which includes functional movement and healthy eating

Community Wellness, which includes belonging and giving back

Mental Wellness, which includes motivation and gratitude

Financial Wellness, which includes financial power and intentional spending

We should pay attention to each of these "pillars" of our lives every day. Sometimes our finances will be the most important; sometimes we'll need to pay special attention to our mental wellness. But if we develop a routine that helps us attend to all these aspects of our lives, most of the time we'll find not perfect balance but a more streamlined, harmonious, and happy way of living.

Fortifying these pillars may seem like a lot to take on, but you don't have to do everything at once. I repeat: You do not have to change everything at the same time. Doing it all is an impossible standard to maintain. You simply need to develop a plan and integrate it, step by step, into your daily routine.

This book is set up using the methodology and framework I use with my coaching clients, delivered at a self-paced, easily consumable, twelve-week format. It focuses on way more than just fitness and physical appearance because, let's be honest, how you look is probably the least interesting thing about you.

To change any aspect of your life, your environment must support your journey to a different lifestyle. One of the best ways to start making changes is to tell those closest to you. Share your intentions with your family and friends, shout it from the rooftop, and then prepare yourself to be held accountable as you work through this program.

THE FOUR PILLARS OF WELLNESS

By shifting your mindset from one of balance to one of integration, it becomes less likely that you will neglect any of the four pillars I mentioned. The problem comes when you don't know how to address each pillar in a real-istic way. No one wakes up each morning and says, "I'm going to integrate my work, self-care, and responsibility perfectly." No matter how well-intentioned we may be, we have only two arms and twenty-four hours in a day. But when we're aware of the structure and priorities in our life, we'll be better positioned to deal with the ups and downs in a positive way.

The only guarantee in life is that nothing is constant, so the best way to start is to accept that and learn to roll with it. Some days, you are going to be a great partner or parent, but you may miss a work deadline or two. Other days, you're going to be a rockstar at your job but you're going to be full of parental guilt. As long as you recognize the shift and don't let things slide too far to the left or right, you are golden!

The same principle applies to your health and well-ness. You aren't going to have it all together every week, but if you recognize the shift toward an extreme, you can make the necessary changes and adjust as needed.

This workbook teaches you how to implement habits, intentions, and reflections into your daily life in a way that can have a positive impact without feeling overwhelming or like a chore. The twelve weeks are designed to build off each other, setting a strong foundation for lasting change.

Each week includes a Week-at-a-Glance calendar, where you can track your habits, plan your days, and keep a high-level overview of what you want to accomplish. This is followed by Daily Plan pages, where you can itemize your to-dos, meal plans, exercise, and water intake. Finally, the week ends with a Weekly Reflection, questions that will help you define and refine your goals and then implement them.

WEEK-AT-A-GLANCE

The Week-at-a-Glance pages are for a quick bird's-eye view of your week. Do you have a big meeting you want to get a good night's sleep for? Write it down. Do you want to try a new fitness class? Jot it down in your movement planner. Are you trying to implement a new habit? Write it down, cross it off, and don't break the chain (see Week 9, page 152). With so much that's digital these days, it's nice to write things on paper if only to give your eyes a break from blue light.

THE DAILY PLAN

The daily planning pages are great for getting more specific about what you want to do each day. By setting your top three priorities, you can avoid trying to do too much in a single day. In Week 2, I discuss Time Blocking and how the Daily Plan can support you in creating and maintaining the Top 3 habit!

WEEKLY REFLECTION

The weekly reflection is an important part of the process. You will reflect on the following four questions each week.

1. *How do you feel about what you accomplished in the last seven days? What went well?*

2. *What do you believe to be the obstacles you faced in accomplishing the goals you set last week?*

3. *What would a "win" look like for this coming week?*

4. *What steps do you need to take to make your "win" a reality?*

Starting off with a win will keep your motivation high and the focus on what's working. You will then reflect on the obstacles you faced. Writing them down will help you keep perspective. We often imagine obstacles to be larger in our heads; seeing them on paper will allow you to stay objective. Next, you envision a win for the upcoming week—an aim as little as getting seven hours of sleep each night or as large as successfully meal prepping for the entire week. Your final question will challenge you to plan the necessary tasks or systems needed to bring your win to fruition. Consider this your accountability tool.

WEEK 1 ·····································

Starting Small

Some plans require you to change everything all at once, but this is not one of those plans. Sudden and drastic changes to your life are not realistic or sustainable. Several studies state that taking on too many changes at once is a recipe for failure.[1] So, we're not going to do that. In fact, we are going to try the complete opposite and start small.

But before I ask you to jump in and start creating your own plan, let me tell you a success story about a client of mine.

Charlotte came to me when she was ready to make a change. As a mother of two young children, she felt that she had lost herself. She didn't recognize her body and had no idea how to get back to some semblance of normalcy. The biggest hurdle was that she hated working out with the passion of a thousand fires.

Where do you start when you have zero desire? Charlotte started with five minutes. We looked at her schedule together and planned two walking days and three workout days. The catch? Her workout days were only five minutes long. Easy, right? You can do anything for five minutes.

After a couple of weeks, five minutes felt too easy, so she increased it to ten minutes. Two weeks later, she increased it to fifteen minutes. Three months later, Charlotte purchased her first set of dumbbells and is now doing full-blown training plans.

While five minutes may not have seemed like a lot at first, using a progressive-overload methodology (setting the foundational habit of movement combined with gradual increases) was the recipe for progress. During this three-month period, Charlotte also paid more attention to her sleep, hydration, and stress levels while tracking them in my coaching app. Once those three basic habits were second nature and I was confident that she would make swift and sustainable progress, we turned our attention to her eating habits.

The struggle and greatest potential for failure happens when we try taking on too many changes at once. If Charlotte had tried to do forty-five minutes of working out, five days a week, I truly believe she would not have been as successful. But by combining things that may be considered easy, with a plan for gradual progressions, she was able to make permanent lifestyle changes.

Focusing on habit formation, paired with a "small changes" approach, has been tested as a behavior change strategy and has been shown to offer an innovative solution for creating lasting health and wellness changes.[2]

As I mention in "The Four Pillars of Wellness" (page 13), the chapters will build off each other and challenge you to take a different approach to everyday life. By making one small change each week, you will create a snowball effect that will build momentum and keep you moving forward.

I encourage you to lean on the resources such as the habit trackers and daily planning pages at the end of each chapter. These are things I find to be helpful when deciding my workouts for the week and my daily "Top 3." You can also use these pages to track any new habits you want to incorporate into your routine.

There's something so fulfilling about checking a box. There is no right or wrong way to set up your week if it works for *you!* If you're unsure how to create a new habit, try the following steps:

HABIT-BUILDING
flow chart

1 Decide on a goal you want to achieve for your health or lifestyle.

2 Choose a simple action that you can do every day.

3 Set a time and place to perform that action. Be consistent.

Walk 10,000 steps a day.

Walk for at least 30 minutes every day.

Every day at 4 p.m. around my neighborhood.

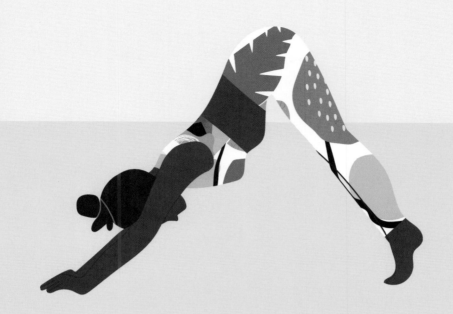

4 Put the plan into action. Be realistic. Don't schedule yourself for a certain time if it turns out you can't do that every day. The key is consistency.

5 It will get easier the more you do it. Within ten weeks, you should find that you are doing the action more intuitively. As you get used to walking every day, start extending the time and distance you walk so you can get closer to that ten-thousand-step goal.

6 Once you are consistently doing your action every day, celebrate the creation of your new habit . . . by starting another healthy habit!

CREATE YOUR OWN
action plan

MY GOAL IS TO

MY PLAN IS TO

(Simple Action) | *(Time & Place)*

I WILL ACHIEVE MY GOAL BY THIS DATE

CELEBRATE THE LITTLE WINS

What is one thing in your life that you are proud of? You may be thinking of something work-related or an educational achievement because big accomplishments are sexy. But what about the little things that got you to those big accomplishments? Those are important too.

"If you want to change the world, start by making your bed."
— *Admiral William H. McRaven*

In Week 2, "Morning Routine" (page 31), I suggest that something as small as making your bed every morning can have a huge impact on the trajectory of your day. It is an accomplishment. It's a small win that's completed first thing in the morning, and if nothing else goes your way that day, you will come home to a freshly made bed. Make your bed and change the world.

Practice

Your first new habit is to get used to planning your days. Resist the urge to start big and add in more changes. Remember, we are taking tiny steps with the goal of making gradual progress.

Set aside time on Sunday afternoons to plan out your week using the Week-at-a-Glance pages!

Week-at-a-Glance

TO-DO LIST

Monday

◯ _____
◯ _____
◯ _____
◯ _____
◯ _____
◯ _____
◯ _____
◯ _____
◯ _____

Tuesday

◯ _____
◯ _____
◯ _____
◯ _____
◯ _____
◯ _____
◯ _____
◯ _____
◯ _____

Wednesday

◯ _____
◯ _____
◯ _____
◯ _____
◯ _____
◯ _____
◯ _____
◯ _____
◯ _____

Habit Tracker

HABIT	M	T	W	Th	F	S	Su

What's for Dinner?

M	
T	
W	
Th	
F	
S	
Su	

___ / ___ / ___ — ___ / ___ /

Thursday

- ○ _____
- ○ _____
- ○ _____
- ○ _____
- ○ _____
- ○ _____
- ○ _____
- ○ _____
- ○ _____

Friday

- ○ _____
- ○ _____
- ○ _____
- ○ _____
- ○ _____
- ○ _____
- ○ _____
- ○ _____
- ○ _____

Saturday

- ○ _____
- ○ _____
- ○ _____
- ○ _____
- ○ _____
- ○ _____
- ○ _____
- ○ _____
- ○ _____

TO-DO LIST

Movement Planner

M	
T	
W	
Th	
F	
S	
Su	

Sunday

- ○ _____
- ○ _____
- ○ _____
- ○ _____
- ○ _____
- ○ _____
- ○ _____
- ○ _____
- ○ _____

TO-DO LIST

Monday

_____ / _____ / _____

Top Priorities

1. _____

2. _____

3. _____

TO-DOS

- ○ _____
- ○ _____
- ○ _____
- ○ _____
- ○ _____
- ○ _____
- ○ _____
- ○ _____
- ○ _____
- ○ _____
- ○ _____

NOTES

MEALS

B	
L	
D	
S	

WATER TRACKER

TIME BLOCKING

:	
:	
:	
:	
:	
:	
:	
:	
:	
:	
:	
:	
:	
:	
:	
:	
:	
:	
:	
:	
:	
:	

_____ / _____ / _____

Tuesday

Top Priorities

1. _____

2. _____

3. _____

MEALS

B	
L	
D	
S	

WATER TRACKER

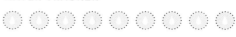

TO-DOS

○ _____
○ _____
○ _____
○ _____
○ _____
○ _____
○ _____
○ _____
○ _____
○ _____
○ _____

TIME BLOCKING

:	
:	
:	
:	
:	
:	
:	
:	
:	
:	
:	
:	
:	
:	
:	
:	
:	
:	
:	
:	

NOTES

Wednesday

_____ / _____ / _____

Top Priorities

1. _____
2. _____
3. _____

TO-DOS

- ○ _____
- ○ _____
- ○ _____
- ○ _____
- ○ _____
- ○ _____
- ○ _____
- ○ _____
- ○ _____
- ○ _____
- ○ _____

NOTES

MEALS

B	
L	
D	
S	

WATER TRACKER

TIME BLOCKING

:	
:	
:	
:	
:	
:	
:	
:	
:	
:	
:	
:	
:	
:	
:	
:	
:	
:	
:	
:	
:	

_____ / _____ / _____

Thursday

Top Priorities

1. _____
2. _____
3. _____

TO-DOS

- _____
- _____
- _____
- _____
- _____
- _____
- _____
- _____
- _____
- _____
- _____

NOTES

MEALS

B	
L	
D	
S	

WATER TRACKER

TIME BLOCKING

:	
:	
:	
:	
:	
:	
:	
:	
:	
:	
:	
:	
:	
:	
:	
:	
:	
:	
:	
:	
:	

Friday

........../........../..........

Top Priorities

1. _____

2. _____

3. _____

TO-DOS

- ○ _____
- ○ _____
- ○ _____
- ○ _____
- ○ _____
- ○ _____
- ○ _____
- ○ _____
- ○ _____
- ○ _____
- ○ _____

NOTES

MEALS

B	
L	
D	
S	

WATER TRACKER

○ ○ ○ ○ ○ ○ ○ ○ ○

TIME BLOCKING

:	
:	
:	
:	
:	
:	
:	
:	
:	
:	
:	
:	
:	
:	
:	
:	
:	
:	
:	
:	
:	
:	

_____ / _____ / _____

Saturday & Sunday

Top Priorities

1. _____
2. _____
3. _____

TO-DOS

- ○ _____
- ○ _____
- ○ _____
- ○ _____
- ○ _____
- ○ _____
- ○ _____
- ○ _____
- ○ _____
- ○ _____
- ○ _____

NOTES

MEALS

B	
L	
D	
S	

WATER TRACKER

○ ○ ○ ○ ○ ○ ○ ○ ○

TIME BLOCKING

:	
:	
:	
:	
:	
:	
:	
:	
:	
:	
:	
:	
:	
:	
:	
:	
:	
:	
:	
:	

WEEKLY REFLECTION

How do you feel about what you accomplished in the last seven days?
What went well?

What do you believe to be the obstacles you faced in accomplishing
the goals you set last week?

What would a "win" look like for this coming week?

What steps do you need to take to make your "win" a reality?

Optimizing Routines & Sleep Hygiene

You've have had some practice planning your weekdays, so let's move on to optimizing your routines, including your sleep hygiene. Routines are so important for babies, but we often forget how important they are for adults. The creation of routines, more specifically family routines, have been linked to the development of social skills and academic success. Adherence to these routines have been shown to aid in resilience during times of stress and crisis and will support not only you but your family as well.

MORNING ROUTINE

As you work to create a morning routine for the majority of your days, consider the following questions:

What is your current morning routine?

_____

_____

_____

_____

_____

_____

_____

_____

Is your current morning routine efficient? Does it support your goals?

_____

_____

_____

_____

_____

_____

_____

_____

If the answer is no, brainstorm some ideas for a new routine. If you answered yes, congratulations, your work is done!

_____

_____

_____

_____

_____

Okay, let's dream a bit. What would your ideal day look like? Don't just list the things you need to do; think about the things you want to do. Would you meditate more? Would you read more? Would you spend more time with your family? How much sleep do you want to get? Write down everything you want to do.

_____

_____

_____

_____

_____

_____

_____

_____

_____

_____

Now that you have your ideal day in mind, what can you do to make it a reality? Start by creating a morning routine that supports your goals. Here are five tips to help you create a morning routine that works for you.

1. Designate a wake-up time and don't hit the snooze button.

2. Keep water by your bed and drink it as soon as you wake.

3. Make your bed—seriously. Even if you don't get anything else done that day, this tiny accomplishment will make you feel good, I promise.

4. Don't look at your phone for the first hour after wake-up.

5. Fill out your Daily Plan, write down three top priorities you want to accomplish for the day, and start with those.

By turning these tips into habits, you're setting yourself up for organized, productive days.

The example on the right shows my current Monday morning routine.

To accomplish my plan, I set my clothes out in the bathroom the night before, keep water by my bed so I can easily grab it and take it with me to the gym, and make sure my evening routine supports an early wakeup.

5:30a	wake up and water
5:45a	30-minute workout and 10-minute stretch
6:30a	coffee, journaling, emails, and content posting
7:00a	wake up kids for school, breakfast, and drop-offs
8:00a	work, play, read until our nanny arrives at 10 a.m.

EVENING ROUTINE

To keep things running smoothly in the evening, I like

4:00p	electronics-free hour with coffee or tea
5:00p	dinner prep
6:00p	dinner with the family around the table
6:45p	play a family game
7:30p	bath and bedtime for the youngest
8:00p	unwind and do a little work
9:30p	nighttime drink
10:00p	book and bed!

to plan dinners in advance. I'm a big believer in meal prep—but I am also not shy about ordering in. My kids know the evening drill, and they always get a fifteen-minute warning. Alexa is our timekeeper: "Alexa, set a timer for fifteen minutes." "Alexa, bathe my children."

The example on the left shows my current evening routine.

Like a morning routine, an evening routine is associated with increased family functioning and improved sleep habits. More importantly, sleep hygiene or lack thereof has been associated with increased stress, decreased cogitative performance, and general lower quality of life. Nearly every key indicator of individual health, such as family well-being, performance, accidents, and injuries, is affected by chronic lack of sleep.

SLEEP HYGIENE

The current culture of our society praises lack of sleep and awards us a badge of honor because we somehow manage the appearance of having it all together. Who is the most exhausted? Who is the busiest? Who has the most Pinterest-worthy home on three-and-a-half hours of sleep? I'm here to say that it's bullshit. Exhausting yourself is not something to be admired.

Once you understand the science behind how lack of sleep affects your hormones and what those hormones are responsible for, I have a feeling you'll work to change your outlook on sleep. Circumstances are one thing, but actively working against your body by pounding gallons of coffee and ignoring your cues is another.

At its core, sleep deprivation is associated with a whole host of physiological changes, ranging from increased inflammation in the body to insulin resistance.[3] Have you ever noticed that your cravings for sweets or salty food increase the day after a terrible night's sleep? That is not a coincidence. Poor sleep leads to an increase in the hunger hormone known as ghrelin. More ghrelin equals more hunger. More hunger equals less than favorable food choices, which can lead to poor sleep, and that turns into a vicious cycle.

Additionally, I'm sure you've noticed that you don't fire on all cylinders after a terrible night of sleep. Sleep deprivation is associated with a decrease in cogitative abilities; that is, your brain doesn't work as well.

How much sleep do I really need?

While this is highly individualized, seven hours is a good baseline for adequate sleep. There are plenty of factors that play into this calculation, such as quality time spent in REM or deep sleep, sleep consistency, and sleep satisfaction. And much like babies, our bodies thrive on routine.

Rather than be a victim of poor sleep routines, create a plan to optimize your rest. A good goal is to go to bed at a consistent time, sleep for approximately seven hours, and wake up at a consistent time. If you recognize that you can't get as much sleep as you would like during the week, add a nap in on the weekends. All sleep matters. With a regular sleep and wake schedule, your body will know when to release calming hormones before bed and stimulating hormones to wake up.

As much as I love a good glass of red, skip the nightly wine-cap and opt for a lavender or chamomile tea instead. Alcohol and coffee can interfere with a restful night's sleep. You should avoid both at least six to eight hours before bedtime.

You can also improve sleep by investing in your sanctuary. Room-darkening curtains can go a long way, and if that isn't an option, a nice silk sleep mask runs a close second. You should also work to declutter your bedroom. Get rid of anything in you room that is causing you stress before bed. This could be piles of clothing that need to be folded or your laptop reminding you that you have a deadline to make in twelve hours. Your bedroom should be a relaxing place of solace, not a constant reminder of what you need to get done.

Lastly, try to work relaxation techniques into your evening. Put electronics away at least an hour before bed. The blue light and distractions are counterproductive to improving sleep hygiene. Take a bath with Epsom salt or add steam tablets to your shower. Aromatherapy is a proven technique as an aid to stress reduction.[4] You can also keep a notepad by your bed. At the end of the night, if your mind is reeling from your to-do list, write it down and let it go until tomorrow. I've found that a brain dump is really effective in freeing up mental capacity. Use that mental capacity to dive into a good novel. Your dreams will thank you!

TIME BLOCKING

You've had some practice creating a new habit, your morning and evening routines are set, but what about the middle of the day? One of the tools I use to help me manage my time is time blocking.

We all have the same twenty-four hours in a day, and roughly seven of those are spent sleeping. That means we have about seventeen hours to spread between work, family, self-care, and everything else. Time blocking involves separating your days into chunks, so you can use your time efficiently and be less likely to

5:00a	
6:00a	
7:00a	*morning routine*
8:00a	
9:00a	*business-focused work*
10:00a	
11:00a	*client-focused work*
12:00p	
1:00p	
2:00p	*creative work*
3:00p	*& movement*
4:00p	
5:00p	
6:00p	
7:00p	*evening routine*
8:00p	
9:00p	
10:00p	

get distracted by tasks that have a lower priority.

You'll notice in the example to the left that my time is separated into chunks with a high-level idea of what I want to accomplish during that time. My morning and evening routines are already defined, therefore they don't deviate from my time-blocked schedule.

I split the middle of my day into two- and three-hour time chunks with a general idea of what I need to accomplish. Studies have shown that your speed and accuracy are both better in the morning, so I suggest planning to do any work that involves critical thinking, such as project tracking or financial planning, first.[5] Get it out of the way while you're fresh and in a favorable mood. Think about it—babies are happiest when they've just woken and are full of milk. Adults are the same way!

"A 40-hour time-blocked work week, I estimate, produces the same amount of output as a 60-plus-hour work week pursued without structure."
—*Cal Newport, author of* Deep Work

I developed the habit of time blocking in 2013 because I was training as a full-time athlete, running a gym, mothering two small children. I had to be efficient, or nothing would get accomplished. I found that when I assigned the tasks to blocks of time, I worked harder to complete them in the time allotted before moving on to the next one.

Try it! You will be less liable to forget to do something and you will be amazed at how productive you are. It's easier to be productive when you know what you must accomplish in small, actionable chunks of time.

Practice

Your turn. Imagine your ideal morning and evening routines. How do you need to arrange your evening routine to ensure that you'll have a good night's rest? How can you make sure to have those things every night?

Practice using Time Blocking in the Daily Plan. Do it every day this week and implement your new routines in the process, making necessary considerations for family scheduling. For example, on Tuesday you might need to pick up the kids from soccer practice and on Thursday you might have a class, so make sure dinner is planned or ordered in for those evenings. By planning for all the little things, you won't need to frantically order food at the last minute or be late picking up your kids. A perk as your life starts to run more smoothly: Your sleep will improve as well.

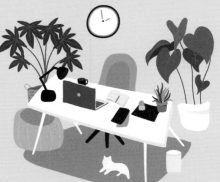

Week-at-a-Glance

TO-DO LIST

Monday

○ _____
○ _____
○ _____
○ _____
○ _____
○ _____
○ _____
○ _____
○ _____

Tuesday

○ _____
○ _____
○ _____
○ _____
○ _____
○ _____
○ _____
○ _____
○ _____

Wednesday

○ _____
○ _____
○ _____
○ _____
○ _____
○ _____
○ _____
○ _____
○ _____

Habit Tracker

HABIT	M	T	W	Th	F	S	Su

What's for Dinner?

M	
T	
W	
Th	
F	
S	
Su	

Thursday

- ⭘ _____
- ⭘ _____
- ⭘ _____
- ⭘ _____
- ⭘ _____
- ⭘ _____
- ⭘ _____
- ⭘ _____
- ⭘ _____

Friday

- ⭘ _____
- ⭘ _____
- ⭘ _____
- ⭘ _____
- ⭘ _____
- ⭘ _____
- ⭘ _____
- ⭘ _____
- ⭘ _____

Saturday

- ⭘ _____
- ⭘ _____
- ⭘ _____
- ⭘ _____
- ⭘ _____
- ⭘ _____
- ⭘ _____
- ⭘ _____
- ⭘ _____

TO-DO LIST

Movement Planner

M	
T	
W	
Th	
F	
S	
Su	

Sunday

- ⭘ _____
- ⭘ _____
- ⭘ _____
- ⭘ _____
- ⭘ _____
- ⭘ _____
- ⭘ _____
- ⭘ _____

TO-DO LIST

Monday

.... / ...... / ....

Top Priorities

1. _____
2. _____
3. _____

TO-DOS

- ○ _____
- ○ _____
- ○ _____
- ○ _____
- ○ _____
- ○ _____
- ○ _____
- ○ _____
- ○ _____
- ○ _____
- ○ _____

NOTES

MEALS

B	
L	
D	
S	

WATER TRACKER

○ ○ ○ ○ ○ ○ ○ ○ ○

TIME BLOCKING

:	
:	
:	
:	
:	
:	
:	
:	
:	
:	
:	
:	
:	
:	
:	
:	
:	
:	
:	
:	
:	

_____ / _____ / _____

Tuesday

Top Priorities

1. _____
2. _____
3. _____

TO-DOS

- ○ _____
- ○ _____
- ○ _____
- ○ _____
- ○ _____
- ○ _____
- ○ _____
- ○ _____
- ○ _____
- ○ _____
- ○ _____

NOTES

MEALS

B	
L	
D	
S	

WATER TRACKER

TIME BLOCKING

:	
:	
:	
:	
:	
:	
:	
:	
:	
:	
:	
:	
:	
:	
:	
:	
:	
:	
:	
:	
:	

Wednesday

.... / ...... / ....

Top Priorities

1. _____
2. _____
3. _____

MEALS

B	
L	
D	
S	

WATER TRACKER

○ ○ ○ ○ ○ ○ ○ ○ ○

TO-DOS

- ○ _____
- ○ _____
- ○ _____
- ○ _____
- ○ _____
- ○ _____
- ○ _____
- ○ _____
- ○ _____
- ○ _____
- ○ _____

TIME BLOCKING

:	
:	
:	
:	
:	
:	
:	
:	
:	
:	
:	
:	
:	
:	
:	
:	
:	
:	
:	
:	
:	

NOTES

.... / .... / ....

Thursday

Top Priorities

1. _____
2. _____
3. _____

TO-DOS

- ○ _____
- ○ _____
- ○ _____
- ○ _____
- ○ _____
- ○ _____
- ○ _____
- ○ _____
- ○ _____
- ○ _____
- ○ _____

NOTES

MEALS

B	
L	
D	
S	

WATER TRACKER

○ ○ ○ ○ ○ ○ ○ ○ ○

TIME BLOCKING

:	
:	
:	
:	
:	
:	
:	
:	
:	
:	
:	
:	
:	
:	
:	
:	
:	
:	
:	
:	
:	

Friday

_____ / _____ / _____

Top Priorities

1. _____
2. _____
3. _____

TO-DOS

- ○ _____
- ○ _____
- ○ _____
- ○ _____
- ○ _____
- ○ _____
- ○ _____
- ○ _____
- ○ _____
- ○ _____
- ○ _____

NOTES

MEALS

B	
L	
D	
S	

WATER TRACKER

TIME BLOCKING

:	
:	
:	
:	
:	
:	
:	
:	
:	
:	
:	
:	
:	
:	
:	
:	
:	
:	
:	
:	
:	

_____ / _____ / _____

Saturday & Sunday

Top Priorities

1. _____
2. _____
3. _____

TO-DOS

- ○ _____
- ○ _____
- ○ _____
- ○ _____
- ○ _____
- ○ _____
- ○ _____
- ○ _____
- ○ _____
- ○ _____
- ○ _____

NOTES

MEALS

B	
L	
D	
S	

WATER TRACKER

○ ○ ○ ○ ○ ○ ○ ○

TIME BLOCKING

:	
:	
:	
:	
:	
:	
:	
:	
:	
:	
:	
:	
:	
:	
:	
:	
:	
:	
:	
:	
:	

WEEKLY REFLECTION

How do you feel about what you accomplished in the last seven days? What went well?

What do you believe to be the obstacles you faced in accomplishing the goals you set last week?

What would a "win" look like for this coming week?

What steps do you need to take to make your "win" a reality?

"If you don't willingly make time for your wellness, you will be forced to make time for your sickness."

—UNKNOWN

Physical Wellness

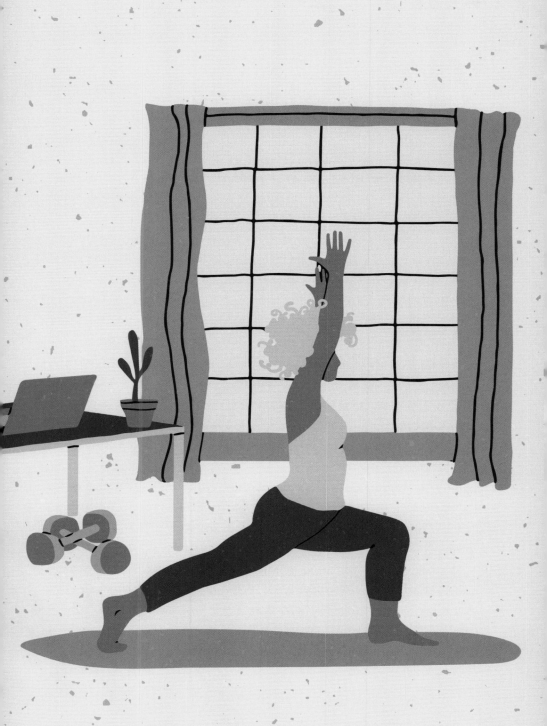

WEEK 3 ··

Movement

My introduction to health and wellness began in 2008 when I stumbled on a video of Eva Twardokens, Annie Sakamoto, and Nicole Carroll doing a CrossFit workout called "Nasty Girls." If you're not familiar with CrossFit, it has several named benchmark workouts. You do one as fast as possible, while maintaining good form. Your score is the time it takes you to complete the workout. Every so often, you retest the workout to gauge your progress in a fitness level. If the amount of time it takes you to do the same workout decreases, you are getting better, faster, stronger.

I was hooked. I wanted to be like Eva, Annie, and Nicole. I wanted to be strong. I dove in headfirst and drank all the CrossFit Kool-Aid. I have since received more CrossFit certifications than I can count. It was during one of those certifications that I first saw this "Sickness/Wellness/Fitness Continuum," and it has stuck with me throughout my career.

Physical health is a lifetime journey, and at any given moment, we can pinpoint each element of our health on the continuum. Ideally, we want to fall somewhere between "wellness" and "fitness."

During my competitive years, I was very close to the Fitness point—I had low levels of body fat, optimal health and blood levels, and peak muscle mass. A few years back, I broke my ankle, which sidelined me for about six weeks. By the end of those six weeks, I had lost five pounds of muscle mass, had gained some fat, and was closer to the "Wellness" point on the continuum. But because I was still very healthy according to the "Sickness/Wellness/Fitness" Continuum, I was able to quickly rebuild. Had I not been as healthy, the impact would've been worse.

For people who are new to fitness, healthy eating, and focusing on their overall wellness, they are going to fall more toward the "Sickness" side of the continuum. This isn't to say that they are sick, but that if they were to become sick or injured, their recovery will likely be more difficult and take longer.

The goal is to get as close to "Fitness" as possible so when you have unexpected or extended periods of downtime, you can minimize the impact to your overall health. Bottom line: Strive to move all aspects of your health and wellness as close to the "Fitness" end of the continuum as possible.

Sickness/Wellness/Fitness Continuum

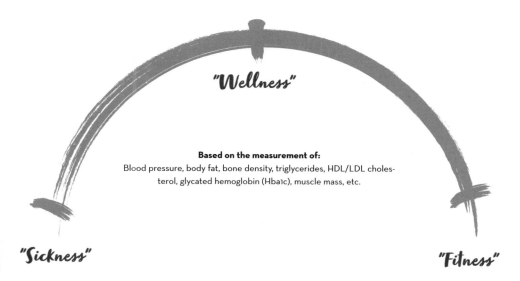

"Wellness"

Based on the measurement of:
Blood pressure, body fat, bone density, triglycerides, HDL/LDL cholesterol, glycated hemoglobin (Hba1c), muscle mass, etc.

"Sickness"

"Fitness"

When was my last physical?

_____

_____

What does health mean to me?

_____

_____

_____

_____

_____

_____

What can I do to impact my physical wellness for the better today?

_____

_____

_____

_____

_____

_____

_____

FUNCTIONAL MOVEMENT

When it comes to movement, I love any exercise that translates to a real-life situation. Drop a cookie on the kitchen floor, the three-second rule applies, so you pick it back up. That's a deadlift. If you fall and stand back up, that's a burpee. When you sit down on the couch and stand back up to grab the remote, that's a squat. See where I'm going? This is called functional movement. Your daily workouts should support the movements you need to use in your daily life.

How much time do I need to spend working out?

The general rule for anyone, as provided by the CDC, is to aim for 30 minutes of movement every day, or 150 minutes each week. If your goal is to lose weight or gain muscle, you will have to increase the time, but this is a good starting point.

During my competitive years, it was completely normal to spend 5 to 6 hours training every day. My days were broken up by coaching, breastfeeding sessions, running a business, and other time-blocked activity.

Today though, I aim to get in 30 to 45 minutes of quality movement, 6 days a week. Combining functional training with a healthy and balanced diet has helped me maintain a level of fitness and body composition that makes me happy.

Notice I said nothing about being at a happy weight. I'm not interested in your weight, because there are plenty of other indicators of a healthy body. Focusing solely on your weight is disrespectful to your blood pressure, body fat, vitamin levels, and hydration—everything that goes into making you *you!* It's incredibly easy to get bogged down by that number, especially because our diet-obsessed culture is difficult to tune out.

Logically speaking, that number is nothing more than your gravitational force on this planet. It is a data point. Nothing more, nothing less. Stop giving it so much power! If tracking that data point makes you uneasy, then don't do it. You work out to be healthy and feel good, not to shrink yourself!

Make sure you check with your doctor or a qualified professional before you adopt a new workout routine to ensure you're healthy enough for physical activity.

MILE A DAY

If you are still having a hard time figuring out how to work movement into your lifestyle, here is something guaranteed to get you moving. Someone I admire very much turned me on to this activity. Commit to running or walking one mile per day. If you are handicapable, rolling one mile is an option. Lasting change comes from continually making the decision to do something different. By dedicating yourself to moving one mile a day, you are challenging yourself to make a different choice. Rather than sitting down after dinner, lace up your shoes and head outdoors.

Start tomorrow. For one month, incorporate a dedicated mile into your daily schedule. You can complete this mile any way you see fit. Walk, crawl, or row (2,000 meters on a rowing machine). At a leisurely walking pace, it may take you 25 minutes, or 8 to 10 minutes at a fast pace. This is a time commitment that isn't cumbersome and is also short enough to include the whole family—even smaller kids. Let's start the momentum and keep it going!

Practice

Start working movement into your lifestyle by implementing a plan to walk one mile every day. Write it into your Daily Plan and check it off on the Habit Tracker in the Week-at-a-Glance every time you complete your mile. Go to the Mark Your Mile form on the following pages and mark an X for every day you complete your mile.

What is your favorite way to move your body?

_____

_____

_____

_____

How many days can you realistically dedicate to working out?

_____

_____

Create a plan to work fitness into your routine. It can be as little as ten minutes a day to start. Short bouts of movement have been shown to be effective in maintaining adherence (see "Starting Small," page 16).

_____

_____

_____

_____

_____

_____

_____

_____

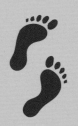

MARK YOUR *mile*

Put an X in the appropriate box for
each day you complete a mile.

	MONDAY	TUESDAY	WEDNESDA
WEEK 1			
WEEK 2			
WEEK 3			
WEEK 4			

THURSDAY	FRIDAY	SATURDAY	SUNDAY

Week-at-a-Glance

TO-DO LIST

Monday
- ○ _____
- ○ _____
- ○ _____
- ○ _____
- ○ _____
- ○ _____
- ○ _____
- ○ _____
- ○ _____

Tuesday
- ○ _____
- ○ _____
- ○ _____
- ○ _____
- ○ _____
- ○ _____
- ○ _____
- ○ _____
- ○ _____

Wednesday
- ○ _____
- ○ _____
- ○ _____
- ○ _____
- ○ _____
- ○ _____
- ○ _____
- ○ _____
- ○ _____

Habit Tracker

HABIT	M	T	W	Th	F	S	Su

What's for Dinner?

M	
T	
W	
Th	
F	
S	
Su	

Thursday

- ○ _____
- ○ _____
- ○ _____
- ○ _____
- ○ _____
- ○ _____
- ○ _____
- ○ _____
- ○ _____

Friday

- ○ _____
- ○ _____
- ○ _____
- ○ _____
- ○ _____
- ○ _____
- ○ _____
- ○ _____
- ○ _____

Saturday

- ○ _____
- ○ _____
- ○ _____
- ○ _____
- ○ _____
- ○ _____
- ○ _____
- ○ _____
- ○ _____

TO-DO LIST

Movement Planner

M	
T	
W	
Th	
F	
S	
Su	

Sunday

- ○ _____
- ○ _____
- ○ _____
- ○ _____
- ○ _____
- ○ _____
- ○ _____
- ○ _____
- ○ _____

TO-DO LIST

Monday

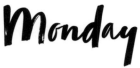

.... / ...... / ....

Top Priorities

1 _____

2 _____

3 _____

TO-DOS

- ○ _____
- ○ _____
- ○ _____
- ○ _____
- ○ _____
- ○ _____
- ○ _____
- ○ _____
- ○ _____
- ○ _____
- ○ _____

NOTES

MEALS

B	
L	
D	
S	

WATER TRACKER

○ ○ ○ ○ ○ ○ ○ ○ ○

TIME BLOCKING

:	
:	
:	
:	
:	
:	
:	
:	
:	
:	
:	
:	
:	
:	
:	
:	
:	
:	
:	
:	
:	
:	

_____ / _____ / _____

Tuesday

Top Priorities

1. _____
2. _____
3. _____

TO-DOS

- ○ _____
- ○ _____
- ○ _____
- ○ _____
- ○ _____
- ○ _____
- ○ _____
- ○ _____
- ○ _____
- ○ _____
- ○ _____

NOTES

MEALS

B	
L	
D	
S	

WATER TRACKER

○ ○ ○ ○ ○ ○ ○ ○ ○

TIME BLOCKING

:	
:	
:	
:	
:	
:	
:	
:	
:	
:	
:	
:	
:	
:	
:	
:	
:	
:	

Wednesday

_____ / _____ / _____

Top Priorities

1. _____
2. _____
3. _____

TO-DOS

- ○ _____
- ○ _____
- ○ _____
- ○ _____
- ○ _____
- ○ _____
- ○ _____
- ○ _____
- ○ _____
- ○ _____

NOTES

MEALS

B	
L	
D	
S	

WATER TRACKER

TIME BLOCKING

:	
:	
:	
:	
:	
:	
:	
:	
:	
:	
:	
:	
:	
:	
:	
:	
:	
:	
:	
:	
:	

_____ / ____ / _____

Thursday

Top Priorities

1. _____
2. _____
3. _____

TO-DOS

- ○ _____
- ○ _____
- ○ _____
- ○ _____
- ○ _____
- ○ _____
- ○ _____
- ○ _____
- ○ _____
- ○ _____
- ○ _____

NOTES

MEALS

B	
L	
D	
S	

WATER TRACKER

○ ○ ○ ○ ○ ○ ○ ○ ○

TIME BLOCKING

:	
:	
:	
:	
:	
:	
:	
:	
:	
:	
:	
:	
:	
:	
:	
:	
:	
:	
:	
:	
:	
:	

Friday

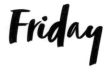

_____ / _____ / _____

Top Priorities

1. _____
2. _____
3. _____

TO-DOS

- ○ _____
- ○ _____
- ○ _____
- ○ _____
- ○ _____
- ○ _____
- ○ _____
- ○ _____
- ○ _____
- ○ _____
- ○ _____

NOTES

MEALS

B	
L	
D	
S	

WATER TRACKER

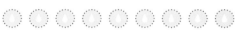

TIME BLOCKING

:	
:	
:	
:	
:	
:	
:	
:	
:	
:	
:	
:	
:	
:	
:	
:	
:	
:	
:	
:	
:	
:	

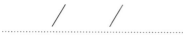

Saturday & Sunday

Top Priorities

1. _____
2. _____
3. _____

TO-DOS

- ○ _____
- ○ _____
- ○ _____
- ○ _____
- ○ _____
- ○ _____
- ○ _____
- ○ _____
- ○ _____
- ○ _____
- ○ _____

NOTES

MEALS

B	
L	
D	
S	

WATER TRACKER

○ ○ ○ ○ ○ ○ ○ ○ ○

TIME BLOCKING

:	
:	
:	
:	
:	
:	
:	
:	
:	
:	
:	
:	
:	
:	
:	
:	
:	
:	
:	
:	

WEEKLY REFLECTION

How do you feel about what you accomplished in the last seven days? What went well?

What do you believe to be the obstacles you faced in accomplishing the goals you set last week?

What would a "win" look like for this coming week?

What steps do you need to take to make your "win" a reality?

WEEK 4 ·······················

Hydration

This week is all about water. Here's a hydration tip from me: Put an 8-ounce glass of water on your bedside table every night before you go to bed. As soon as you wake up, drink it. This will set you up to continue hydrating for the rest of the day.

In the United States, approximately 75 percent of the population suffers from chronic dehydration.[6] We're all familiar with the common symptoms of dehydration such as dry lips, dry mouth, and thirst, but do you know the other symptoms?

The definition of dehydration is a decrease in total body water content due to lack of fluid intake, fluid loss, or both. Beyond making you feel dry and thirsty, dehydration can also cause muscle fatigue, lack of focus, headaches, and general weakness. A human can live for only approximately four days without water.

Our bodies are 70 percent water, and it is vital to our daily functions. It helps us regulate body temperature, aids in digestion, balances oxygen levels, and so much more, so it's important to hydrate regularly and consistently. If you're thirsty, you're already dehydrated. According to the Mayo Clinic, by the time thirst kicks in, you've already lost 1 to 2 percent of your body's water.

All fluids count toward your daily water intake, except for alcohol. This means that your spiked tonic water doesn't count. Alcoholic beverages are a diuretic, and they will decrease your hydration, not increase it. For optimum hydration, stick to water, tea, and coffee.

HOW MUCH IS ENOUGH?

How much water do I actually need to consume?

This helpful hydration formula will guide you! Keep in mind that dehydration sends the same signal as hunger. If you feel hungry, try drinking some water before you head to the pantry.

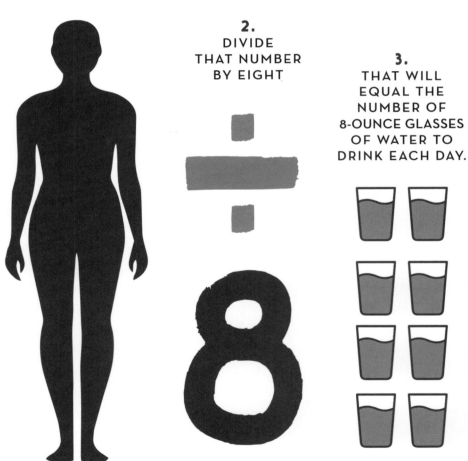

1.
DIVIDE YOUR
BODY WEIGHT
IN HALF

2.
DIVIDE
THAT NUMBER
BY EIGHT

3.
THAT WILL
EQUAL THE
NUMBER OF
8-OUNCE GLASSES
OF WATER TO
DRINK EACH DAY.

That's a lot of glasses of water. But there are other ways you can achieve your hydration goal.

You can eat your way there. Many fruits and vegetables have a high-water composition. For example, watermelon is 92 percent water and tomatoes are 95 percent water. Mixing in fruits and veggies will help you get to your minimum water goal. Go to the next page for the top 10 hydrating foods.

What is the easiest way to tell if I'm hydrated?

On your journey to optimal hydration, you'll be spending more time in the bathroom until your body adjusts. While you're in there, take a peek and see what color your urine is. If it's closer to the color of apple juice, you're dehydrated. If it's closer to the color of watered-down lemonade, congratulations. You're hydrated!

Practice

Based on the hydration formula, calculate how many 8-ounce glasses of water you should be drinking each day. If the number is strikingly high, start with 50 percent of that goal and add 8 ounces of water to your daily goal each week. Rome was not built in a day, and neither will your hydration habit. The Daily Plan has a section to help you track your water intake. Use it to develop the habit of proper hydration.

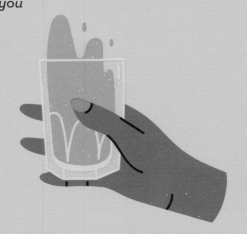

TOP 10
hydrating foods

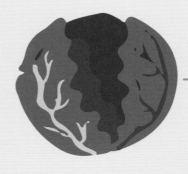

LETTUCE
96%

BLUEBERRIES
95%

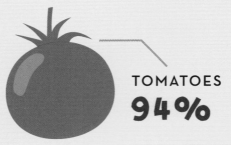

TOMATOES
94%

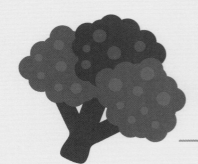

BROCCOLI
92%

CANTALOUPE
92%

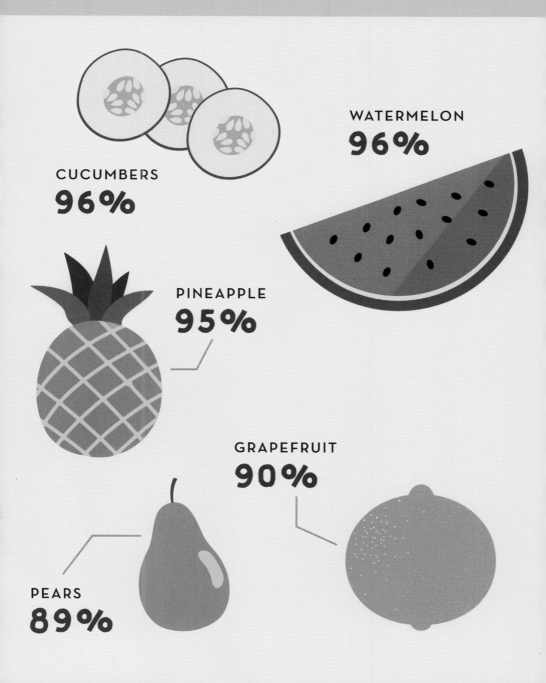

CUCUMBERS
96%

WATERMELON
96%

PINEAPPLE
95%

GRAPEFRUIT
90%

PEARS
89%

Week-at-a-Glance

TO-DO LIST

Monday
- ○ _____
- ○ _____
- ○ _____
- ○ _____
- ○ _____
- ○ _____
- ○ _____
- ○ _____
- ○ _____

Tuesday
- ○ _____
- ○ _____
- ○ _____
- ○ _____
- ○ _____
- ○ _____
- ○ _____
- ○ _____
- ○ _____

Wednesday
- ○ _____
- ○ _____
- ○ _____
- ○ _____
- ○ _____
- ○ _____
- ○ _____
- ○ _____
- ○ _____

Habit Tracker

HABIT	M	T	W	Th	F	S	Su

What's for Dinner?

M	
T	
W	
Th	
F	
S	
Su	

Thursday

- ○ _____
- ○ _____
- ○ _____
- ○ _____
- ○ _____
- ○ _____
- ○ _____
- ○ _____
- ○ _____

Friday

- ○ _____
- ○ _____
- ○ _____
- ○ _____
- ○ _____
- ○ _____
- ○ _____
- ○ _____
- ○ _____

Saturday

- ○ _____
- ○ _____
- ○ _____
- ○ _____
- ○ _____
- ○ _____
- ○ _____
- ○ _____
- ○ _____

TO-DO LIST

Movement Planner

M	
T	
W	
Th	
F	
S	
Su	

Sunday

- ○ _____
- ○ _____
- ○ _____
- ○ _____
- ○ _____
- ○ _____
- ○ _____
- ○ _____

TO-DO LIST

Monday

...... / ...... / ......

Top Priorities

1. _____
2. _____
3. _____

TO-DOS

- ○ _____
- ○ _____
- ○ _____
- ○ _____
- ○ _____
- ○ _____
- ○ _____
- ○ _____
- ○ _____
- ○ _____
- ○ _____

NOTES

MEALS

B	
L	
D	
S	

WATER TRACKER

○ ○ ○ ○ ○ ○ ○ ○ ○

TIME BLOCKING

:	
:	
:	
:	
:	
:	
:	
:	
:	
:	
:	
:	
:	
:	
:	
:	
:	
:	
:	
:	
:	
:	

Tuesday

...... / ...... / ......

Top Priorities

1. _____
2. _____
3. _____

TO-DOS

- ○ _____
- ○ _____
- ○ _____
- ○ _____
- ○ _____
- ○ _____
- ○ _____
- ○ _____
- ○ _____
- ○ _____
- ○ _____

NOTES

MEALS

B	
L	
D	
S	

WATER TRACKER

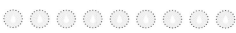

TIME BLOCKING

:	
:	
:	
:	
:	
:	
:	
:	
:	
:	
:	
:	
:	
:	
:	
:	
:	
:	
:	
:	
:	

Wednesday

_____ / _____ / _____

Top Priorities

1. _____
2. _____
3. _____

TO-DOS

○ _____
○ _____
○ _____
○ _____
○ _____
○ _____
○ _____
○ _____
○ _____
○ _____
○ _____

NOTES

MEALS

B	
L	
D	
S	

WATER TRACKER

TIME BLOCKING

:	
:	
:	
:	
:	
:	
:	
:	
:	
:	
:	
:	
:	
:	
:	
:	
:	
:	
:	
:	
:	
:	

Thursday

_____ / _____ / _____

Top Priorities

1. _____
2. _____
3. _____

TO-DOS

- ○ _____
- ○ _____
- ○ _____
- ○ _____
- ○ _____
- ○ _____
- ○ _____
- ○ _____
- ○ _____
- ○ _____
- ○ _____

NOTES

MEALS

B	
L	
D	
S	

WATER TRACKER

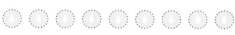

TIME BLOCKING

:	
:	
:	
:	
:	
:	
:	
:	
:	
:	
:	
:	
:	
:	
:	
:	
:	
:	
:	
:	

Friday

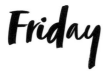

.... / .... / ....

Top Priorities

1. _____

2. _____

3. _____

TO-DOS

- ○ _____
- ○ _____
- ○ _____
- ○ _____
- ○ _____
- ○ _____
- ○ _____
- ○ _____
- ○ _____
- ○ _____
- ○ _____

NOTES

MEALS

B	
L	
D	
S	

WATER TRACKER

TIME BLOCKING

:	
:	
:	
:	
:	
:	
:	
:	
:	
:	
:	
:	
:	
:	
:	
:	
:	
:	
:	
:	
:	

_____ / _____ / _____

Saturday & Sunday

Top Priorities

1. _____
2. _____
3. _____

TO-DOS

- ○ _____
- ○ _____
- ○ _____
- ○ _____
- ○ _____
- ○ _____
- ○ _____
- ○ _____
- ○ _____
- ○ _____
- ○ _____

NOTES

MEALS

B	
L	
D	
S	

WATER TRACKER

○ ○ ○ ○ ○ ○ ○ ○ ○

TIME BLOCKING

:	
:	
:	
:	
:	
:	
:	
:	
:	
:	
:	
:	
:	
:	
:	
:	
:	
:	
:	
:	
:	
:	

WEEKLY REFLECTION

How do you feel about what you accomplished in the last seven days? What went well?

What do you believe to be the obstacles you faced in accomplishing the goals you set last week?

What would a "win" look like for this coming week?

What steps do you need to take to make your "win" a reality?

WEEK 5

Eating with Intention

Growing up, you probably heard the saying "An apple a day keeps the doctor away." Of course, it's not totally true, but how do you go from having this high-level idea of nutrition to implementing a healthy diet into your lifestyle with a goal of optimal health? You start with the basics!

The phrase "counting macros" is often used in conversations around healthy eating, but do you know what macros are exactly? The term *macros* is short for *macronutrients*—units of protein, carbohydrates, and fat—the nutrients your body needs in large amounts. In order to understand macros, you need an introductory understanding of calories (units of energy), as macros are calories and calories are macros. They are what your body runs on.

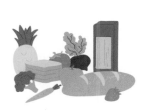 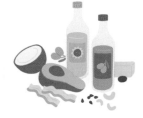 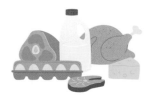

| **CARBOHYDRATES** | **FATS** | **PROTEIN** |
| 1 GRAM = 4 CALORIES | 1 GRAM = 9 CALORIES | 1 GRAM = 4 CALORIES |

TOP PROTEIN
Sources

Beans
16g protein/cup

Cooked Lentils
16g protein/cup

Hard Cheese
7g protein/gram

Cottage Cheese
28g protein/cup

Greek Yogurt
23g protein/cup

Green Peas
8g protein/cup

Hemp seeds
64g protein/cup

Chia Seeds
48g protein/cup

Edamame
20g protein/cup

Almonds
48g protein/cup

Peanut Butter
58g protein/cup

Quinoa
8g protein/cup

Eggs
6g protein/large egg

Grilled Salmon
22g protein/100 grams

Lean Chicken
28g protein/100 grams

Are macros really that important? Yes and no. When you are just beginning to rethink your diet, always remember: quality of food over quantity of food! This means you're better off including unlimited veggies in your diet than worrying about counting the macros of those veggies.

However, if you are farther along in your fitness journey, macros matter. Most weight-loss goals are a simple math problem.

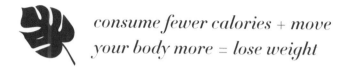

consume fewer calories + move your body more = lose weight

Nutrition is not one size fits all. If someone is trying to sell you a quick-fix guide to shed the pounds, run the other way. My coaching methodology focuses more on strengthening your bond with food, not restricting it. The more you know about what you're eating, the more you can control it.

I don't believe in permanently eliminating foods from your diet unless you have a medical need. I prefer to use the 80/20 method, which encourages people to become intuitive eaters who don't fear certain food groups. The idea is to eat well-balanced meals 80 percent of the time and treat yourself 20 percent of the time. For example, if you eat 10 meals in two days, 8 of those will contain a healthy balance of protein, carbs, and fat. The other 2 meals might include pizza or a peanut butter and chocolate candy that rhymes with *pieces*. This may mean that you'll achieve any of your weight-loss goals slower, but you'll be happier for it. Six-pack abs are not worth the lifestyle trade-off, in my opinion. It's important to choose a diet that supports your lifestyle and goals.

Any nutrition coach will tell you that, like any relationship, your relationship with food should be one of intention and positivity, not one of anxiety and fear. On page 87 is a very simple food-tracking form I use with my clients.

You write down not only what you're eating but how you feel when you're eating it. It's a really good way to home in on your emotions tied to eating. Maybe you'll discover that you eat when you're not even hungry. Watching your eating habits can help you identify and change any unfavorable patterns and potentially address them with a qualified professional.

Practice

Track everything you eat for five days and be honest with your thoughts and feelings. Once you can identify low-hanging fruit, such as late-night snacking out of boredom, you can work to adjust. For example, I discovered that I eat chocolate when I'm bored and have a bad habit of skipping meals unintentionally. In response, I now trade chocolate for fruit and plan lunch so I'll eat it. This helps me make room for the things I truly love, like my apple crumble pie (page 120)!

At the end of the five days, find one habit to change for the better and implement it. Continue adding a new change each week until you reach a point where your diet fits your ideal lifestyle. And if you have no idea what kind of lifestyle you want to live, keep reading. The centenarians of the Blue Zones (page 98) seem to have found the sweet spot!

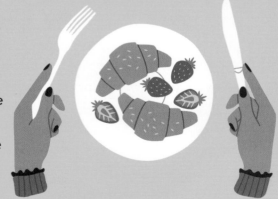

sample FOOD & ACTIVITY TRACKER

TIME	FOOD & DRINK (TYPE & AMOUNT)	PHYSICAL SYMPTOMS, THOUGHTS, FEELINGS	AM I HUNGRY?
7:30a	2 pieces of toast with butter, 2 cups of coffee	I was running late, so I grabbed something quick	Yes
9:30a	1/2 banana, 1 container of blueberry yogurt	In between meetings at work, I wanted to eat something light.	Somewhat
12:30p	2 slices of pepperoni pizza, a side of garden salad with Italian dressing, 1 bottled water	Growling stomach, I was starved! It was a great break from work	Yes!
3:30p	1 can of diet cola, a small bowl of chips with salsa and cheese dip	A co-worker brought a treat for everyone, I just had to sample it.	Not really
7:00p	1 grilled chicken breast, 1 baked potato with 2 spoonfuls of sour cream and 1 spoonful of margarine, 1 helping of broccoli, 1 brownie square, 2 glasses of iced tea	After playing outside for a bit with the kids, I was definitely ready to eat.	Yes
9:00p	2 oatmeal raisin cookies with a glass of 2% milk	I was craving something sweet.	Sort of

DATE ___ / ___ / ___

TIME	FOOD & DRINK (TYPE & AMOUNT)	PHYSICAL SYMPTOMS, THOUGHTS, FEELINGS	AM I HUNGRY?

DATE .... / .... / ....

TIME	FOOD & DRINK (TYPE & AMOUNT)	PHYSICAL SYMPTOMS, THOUGHTS, FEELINGS	AM I HUNGRY?

DATE ___ / ___ / ___

TIME	FOOD & DRINK (TYPE & AMOUNT)	PHYSICAL SYMPTOMS, THOUGHTS, FEELINGS	AM I HUNGRY?

DATE _____ / _____ / _____

TIME	FOOD & DRINK (TYPE & AMOUNT)	PHYSICAL SYMPTOMS, THOUGHTS, FEELINGS	AM I HUNGRY?

DATE ____ / ____ / ____

TIME	FOOD & DRINK (TYPE & AMOUNT)	PHYSICAL SYMPTOMS, THOUGHTS, FEELINGS	AM I HUNGRY?

DATE .... / ...... / ....

TIME	FOOD & DRINK (TYPE & AMOUNT)	PHYSICAL SYMPTOMS, THOUGHTS, FEELINGS	AM I HUNGRY?

WEEKLY REFLECTION

How do you feel about what you accomplished in the last seven days? What went well?

What do you believe to be the obstacles you faced in accomplishing the goals you set last week?

What would a "win" look like for this coming week?

What steps do you need to take to make your "win" a reality?

"Alone we
can do so little;
together we can
do so much!"

-HELEN KELLER

PILLAR II

Community Wellness

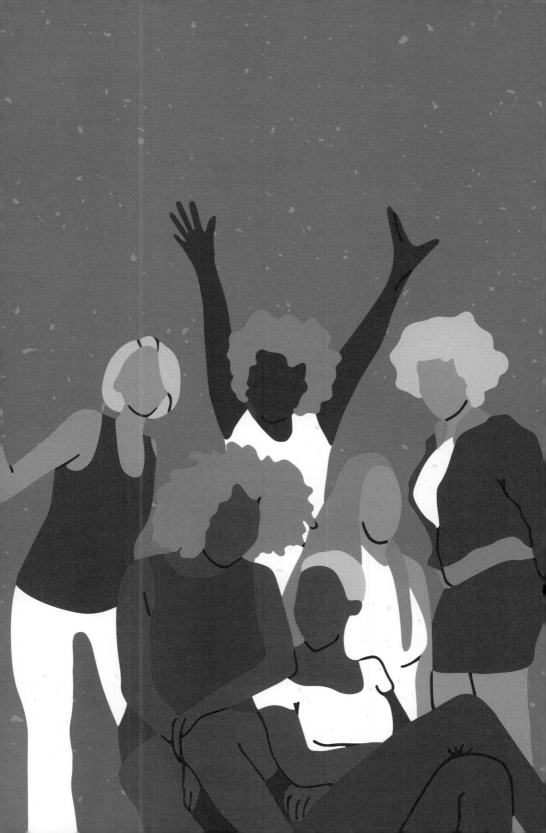

WEEK 6 ·····································

Blue Zones

Recently our family watched all the episodes of the documentary show *Down to Earth with Zac Efron*. If you haven't seen it, go there now. That's where I first learned the term *Blue Zone*. Blue Zone is a nonscientific term coined by National Geographic Fellow Dan Buettner to describe geographic regions that are home to some of the world's oldest people.

Buettner and his team isolated five locations that met their research criteria:

Okinawa, Japan
Nicola, Costa Rica
Loma Linda, California
Sardinia, Italy
Icaria, Greece

What is it about these places that make their populations live so long? Dan and his team narrowed it down to the following nine factors:

1. They move naturally. The world's longest-lived people don't spend hours in the gym or run marathons. They live in an environment that is conducive to constant movement throughout the day. They walk instead of drive, they work in their gardens, and they rely very little on mechanical conveniences. The movement comes naturally.

2. They have defined their purpose. The Okinawans call it *ikigai* and the Nicoyans call it *plan de vida*. This purpose is the reason to wake up in the morning. The people that live in Blue Zones have a sense of purpose. Knowing your sense of purpose adds up to seven extra years of life expectancy.

3. They understand the role stress plays on their bodies. Stress is known to cause chronic inflammation, which is associated with every age-related disease. People in the Blue Zones take a few moments out of every day to pray, meditate, or just be. This is a tool all of us could implement to decrease stress naturally.

4. They live by the 80 percent rule. In Okinawa it's called *hara hachi bu*, and it's a 2,500-year-old Confucian mantra that is said before meals to remind them to stop eating when they are 80 percent full. That remaining 20 percent is the difference between gaining weight and losing it. Most people in the Blue Zones eat their smallest meal at the end of the day and don't eat again until the following morning.

5. Blue Zone inhabitants rely more on vegetables than meat. When they do eat meat, it is maybe five times per month, not every day. Beans make up the majority of most centenarian diets.

6. People in the Blue Zones drink alcohol regularly, but moderately. The trick is to drink only one to two glasses per day, with friends or with food. Drinking alone on your couch while binging mindless TV does not count.

7. The majority of centenarians that Buettner interviewed belonged to some kind of faith-based community. Denomination doesn't seem to matter. Research shows that attending faith-based services four times per month will add four to fourteen years of life expectancy.

8. People who live in the Blue Zones put their families first. Their aging parents live nearby, they commit to a life partner, and they shower their children with love and quality time. This focus can add years to your life and lower mortality rates.

9. Those in the Blue Zone choose to surround themselves with social circles that support healthy behaviors. Research from the Framingham Heart Study shows that smoking, obesity, happiness, and even loneliness is contagious. A social circle that values the same lifestyle choices is vitally important for overall health.

Why am I telling you all this? Because people often assume the secret to living a healthy and happy life comes in a quick seven-day cleanse or a new thirty-day challenge. It doesn't. It comes from moving your body more, being mindful of your food intake, and practicing gratitude, mixed with a little faith. Rather than spinning a globe and dropping your finger on your new home in search of longevity, look inward and create your own Blue Zone.

Practice

Implement one of the nine Blue Zone principles into your life and journal about it each day (for tips on how to journal, see page 153).

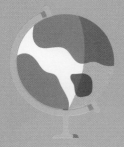

We can't all go and live in a Blue Zone, but we can implement some of their habits. Which of the nine factors of Blue Zone longevity can you implement into your own life where you live right now?

_____

_____

_____

_____

_____

_____

_____

_____

_____

_____

_____

_____

_____

_____

_____

_____

_____

_____

What is your purpose or reason for getting up in the morning? Does it fulfill you?

_____

_____

_____

_____

_____

_____

_____

How can you downshift more intentionally? What steps can you take to unplug and avoid always being "on"? Maybe blocking email or social media from your phone on the weekends?

_____

_____

_____

_____

_____

_____

_____

Do you drink alcohol? Do you think you drink more than you should? Try limiting your alcohol intake this week to one glass per day and see how you feel.

_____

_____

_____

Does your social circle support a healthy lifestyle? If not, what steps can you take to change that?

_____

_____

_____

_____

_____

_____

_____

_____

_____

_____

_____

_____

_____

Week-at-a-Glance

TO-DO LIST

Monday

- ⃝ _____
- ⃝ _____
- ⃝ _____
- ⃝ _____
- ⃝ _____
- ⃝ _____
- ⃝ _____
- ⃝ _____
- ⃝ _____

Tuesday

- ⃝ _____
- ⃝ _____
- ⃝ _____
- ⃝ _____
- ⃝ _____
- ⃝ _____
- ⃝ _____
- ⃝ _____
- ⃝ _____

Wednesday

- ⃝ _____
- ⃝ _____
- ⃝ _____
- ⃝ _____
- ⃝ _____
- ⃝ _____
- ⃝ _____
- ⃝ _____
- ⃝ _____

Habit Tracker

HABIT	M	T	W	Th	F	S	Su

What's for Dinner?

M	
T	
W	
Th	
F	
S	
Su	

Thursday

- ◯ _____
- ◯ _____
- ◯ _____
- ◯ _____
- ◯ _____
- ◯ _____
- ◯ _____
- ◯ _____
- ◯ _____

Friday

- ◯ _____
- ◯ _____
- ◯ _____
- ◯ _____
- ◯ _____
- ◯ _____
- ◯ _____
- ◯ _____
- ◯ _____

Saturday

- ◯ _____
- ◯ _____
- ◯ _____
- ◯ _____
- ◯ _____
- ◯ _____
- ◯ _____
- ◯ _____
- ◯ _____

TO-DO LIST

Movement Planner

M	
T	
W	
Th	
F	
S	
Su	

Sunday

- ◯ _____
- ◯ _____
- ◯ _____
- ◯ _____
- ◯ _____
- ◯ _____
- ◯ _____
- ◯ _____
- ◯ _____

TO-DO LIST

Monday

_____ / _____ / _____

Top Priorities

1. _____
2. _____
3. _____

TO-DOS

- ○ _____
- ○ _____
- ○ _____
- ○ _____
- ○ _____
- ○ _____
- ○ _____
- ○ _____
- ○ _____
- ○ _____
- ○ _____

NOTES

MEALS

B	
L	
D	
S	

WATER TRACKER

TIME BLOCKING

:	
:	
:	
:	
:	
:	
:	
:	
:	
:	
:	
:	
:	
:	
:	
:	
:	
:	
:	
:	
:	

_____ / _____ / _____

Tuesday

Top Priorities

1. _____
2. _____
3. _____

TO-DOS

- ○ _____
- ○ _____
- ○ _____
- ○ _____
- ○ _____
- ○ _____
- ○ _____
- ○ _____
- ○ _____
- ○ _____
- ○ _____

NOTES

MEALS

B	
L	
D	
S	

WATER TRACKER

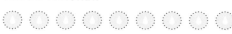

TIME BLOCKING

:	
:	
:	
:	
:	
:	
:	
:	
:	
:	
:	
:	
:	
:	
:	
:	
:	
:	
:	
:	
:	

Wednesday

.... / .... / ....

Top Priorities

1. _____
2. _____
3. _____

TO-DOS

- _____
- _____
- _____
- _____
- _____
- _____
- _____
- _____
- _____
- _____
- _____

NOTES

MEALS

B	
L	
D	
S	

WATER TRACKER

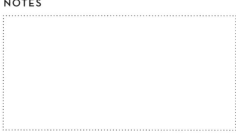

TIME BLOCKING

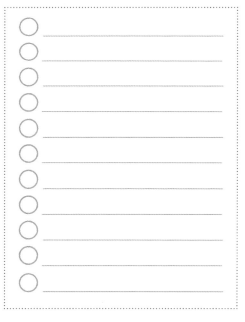

_____ / _____ / _____

Thursday

Top Priorities

1. _____
2. _____
3. _____

TO-DOS

- ○ _____
- ○ _____
- ○ _____
- ○ _____
- ○ _____
- ○ _____
- ○ _____
- ○ _____
- ○ _____
- ○ _____
- ○ _____

NOTES

MEALS

B	
L	
D	
S	

WATER TRACKER

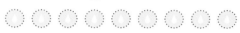

TIME BLOCKING

:	
:	
:	
:	
:	
:	
:	
:	
:	
:	
:	
:	
:	
:	
:	
:	
:	
:	
:	
:	
:	

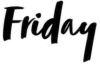

Friday

_____/_____/_____

Top Priorities

1. _____
2. _____
3. _____

TO-DOS

- ○ _____
- ○ _____
- ○ _____
- ○ _____
- ○ _____
- ○ _____
- ○ _____
- ○ _____
- ○ _____
- ○ _____
- ○ _____

NOTES

MEALS

B	
L	
D	
S	

WATER TRACKER

○ ○ ○ ○ ○ ○ ○ ○ ○

TIME BLOCKING

:	
:	
:	
:	
:	
:	
:	
:	
:	
:	
:	
:	
:	
:	
:	
:	
:	
:	
:	
:	
:	
:	

_____ / _____ / _____

Saturday & Sunday

Top Priorities

1. _____
2. _____
3. _____

TO-DOS

- ○ _____
- ○ _____
- ○ _____
- ○ _____
- ○ _____
- ○ _____
- ○ _____
- ○ _____
- ○ _____
- ○ _____

NOTES

MEALS

B	
L	
D	
S	

WATER TRACKER

○ ○ ○ ○ ○ ○ ○ ○ ○ ○

TIME BLOCKING

:	
:	
:	
:	
:	
:	
:	
:	
:	
:	
:	
:	
:	
:	
:	
:	
:	
:	
:	
:	
:	

WEEKLY REFLECTION

How do you feel about what you accomplished in the last seven days? What went well?

What do you believe to be the obstacles you faced in accomplishing the goals you set last week?

What would a "win" look like for this coming week?

What steps do you need to take to make your "win" a reality?

WEEK 7 ··

Mindful Nutrition

FOOD IS MORE THAN JUST FUEL!

In the health and wellness industry, you often hear that "food is just fuel." Quite frankly, that phrase is bullshit. Unless you are a high-level athlete, paid to train full time, food is way more than just fuel. Food is cultural, it provides comfort, and on some days, it's an experience.

When my daughters make enchiladas with their grandmother and learn the recipes, it is cultural; it enhances their connection to the food and to their family. When I made apple pie after my miscarriage, it gave me comfort and still does. Every year we visit the same restaurant for my husband's birthday, a tradition that we love and look forward to. Food is all these things and more. It's meant to be enjoyed, not a punishment to shrink your body. If you look to the Blue Zone inhabitants for inspiration, you will notice that they enjoy their meals, eating slowly, speaking fast, and spending time with those they love.

When you remove the self-imposed mindset and strict rules around food, you will notice a shift. It's often assumed that because

I work in the wellness industry, I have a perfect diet, and maybe I do, because I eat foods that sound good, nourish my body, and make me happy.

Most days, food is just food, a necessity for life. On those occasions when you just need to keep bellies full, it's okay to keep things simple and lean on your meal-prepping skills to get you through the mundane.

MEAL PREP

In my world, meal prep means cooking food in bulk so you have something easy to grab during the week.

For example, on Sunday you might cook two chicken breasts and 1 pound of ground beef. Wash and dry a couple of heads of lettuce. Prepare 4 to 6 cups of rice. Chop up fresh fruits and vegetables. Store them all in glass airtight containers in the refrigerator, and you'll have the basics ready for meals throughout the week. And you'll be less inclined to call for takeout, where you have little control over what goes into the dishes.

For easy consumption, rather than weighing and measuring your food, I want to introduce you to a method that has been taught for years throughout the nutrition community. It's called the "hand portion" method because you use your own hand to determine the amount of a single portion of protein, vegetables, carbohydrates, and fats.

I like this method because weighing your food might not always be an available or interesting option. Perhaps you're at a restaurant or a party. By measuring against your hand, you'll be able to estimate a healthy portion size and avoid overeating. No one likes that stuffed-to-the-brim, I-shouldn't-have-had-that-last-serving feeling.

On any given night, I usually can be found feeding four to six hungry mouths, and they all have different demands. I'm going to be honest: Dinnertime is my least favorite time of day if I have to do the cooking. That's why I decided to plan a weekly menu. I ensure that each meal includes something that everyone will eat. If you're truly hungry, you will be satisfied. To get started, try one of my favorite recipes, Baked Lemon-Butter Chicken (page 233). The bonus is that it requires very little effort.

The Hand Portion Method

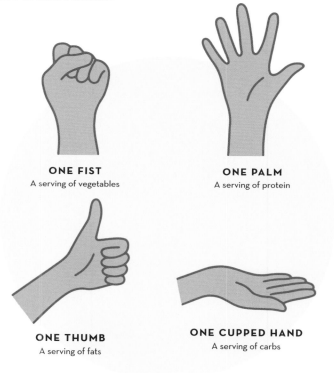

ONE FIST
A serving of vegetables

ONE PALM
A serving of protein

ONE THUMB
A serving of fats

ONE CUPPED HAND
A serving of carbs

Practice

Try your hand at planning meals (use my healthy shopping lists in Resources as a cheat sheet.) Start with Monday, Wednesday, and Friday so you don't get too overwhelmed. As the weeks go by, you can add more days.

MENU *planning*

MONDAY

BREAKFAST	LUNCH	DINNER

TUESDAY

BREAKFAST	LUNCH	DINNER

WEDNESDAY

BREAKFAST	LUNCH	DINNER

THURSDAY

BREAKFAST	LUNCH	DINNER

FRIDAY

BREAKFAST	LUNCH	DINNER

SATURDAY

BREAKFAST	LUNCH	DINNER

SUNDAY

BREAKFAST	LUNCH	DINNER

MONDAY

BREAKFAST	LUNCH	DINNER

TUESDAY

BREAKFAST	LUNCH	DINNER

WEDNESDAY

BREAKFAST	LUNCH	DINNER

THURSDAY

BREAKFAST	LUNCH	DINNER

FRIDAY

BREAKFAST	LUNCH	DINNER

SATURDAY

BREAKFAST	LUNCH	DINNER

SUNDAY

BREAKFAST	LUNCH	DINNER

My Love Affair
WITH
Apple Pie

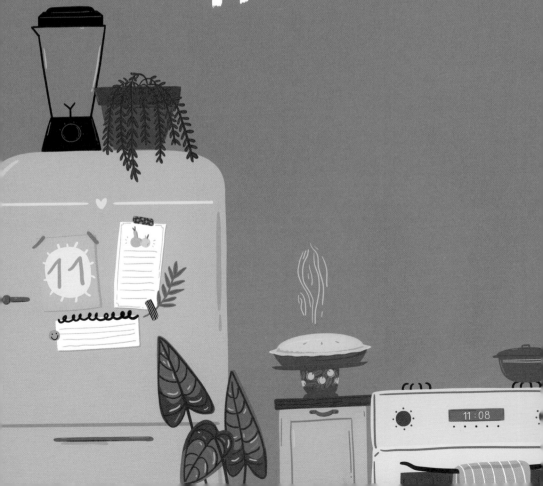

Now that all the serious stuff is out of the way, I am going to grace you with my famous apple pie recipe for no other reason than because I love it!

My love affair with apple pie runs deep. It was the only thing I could stomach during my second pregnancy, and I attribute its magical qualities to my optimal weight gain! However, we all have those moments during pregnancy that we're not necessarily proud of. This is mine: I distinctly remember a day during that pregnancy, when we had only one slice of pie remaining. I left it in the oven, nestled safely in its pie pan. When I heard that distinct sound of the oven door creak from the next room, I knew what was happening. My husband was after my pie. It was like some hormonal, demonic creature took over my body and I exclaimed, "I will cut you if you eat that last slice!" Needless to say, he put my pie back and escaped certain death.

On the hunt for the perfect pie recipe, I found and adapted this one a few years ago. The crumble is particularly amazing.

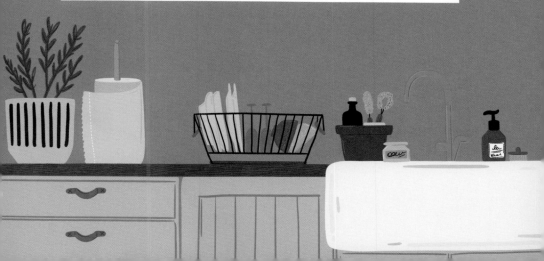

APPLE CRUMBLE PIE

For the crust

3 cups organic
unbleached
all-purpose flour,
plus more for rolling

1 cup butter,
chilled and cubed

1 large egg

2 teaspoons apple
cider vinegar

1 teaspoon sea salt

½ cup room
temperature water

For the filling

6 apples, peeled, cored,
and sliced (I use 3 green
and 3 red)

1½ tablespoons
lemon juice

⅓ cup brown sugar

⅓ cup granulated sugar

¼ cup organic
unbleached
all-purpose flour

1 teaspoon
ground cinnamon

For the crumble topping

1 cup organic
unbleached
all-purpose flour

⅓ cup brown sugar

⅓ cup granulated sugar

½ cup butter,
chilled and cubed

Preheat the oven to 375°F. Place the oven rack in the lowest position. Have ready a 9-inch pie plate.

To make the crust

In a large bowl, mix the flour, butter, egg, vinegar, and salt. Add the water—I usually start with a with ½ cup and add a little more until the dough is no longer sticky. Form it into a ball, cover with plastic wrap, and refrigerate for at least 30 minutes.

Roll out the dough so it will fit on the 9-inch pie plate. Place in the refrigerator while you make the filling.

To make the filling

In a large bowl, combine the apples, lemon juice, brown sugar, granulated sugar, flour, and cinnamon and toss until well combined. Set aside.

To make the topping

In a medium bowl, combine the flour, brown sugar, granulated sugar, and butter. Using your hands, squeeze the ingredients together until the mixture is crumbly. This takes some patience and self-control to stop yourself from eating the crumbles as you form them.

To assemble

Remove the pie plate from the refrigerator. Spoon the apple filling into the crust and spread it out evenly. You can discard any liquid in the bowl.

Sprinkle the crumble topping evenly over the apples. Using a sharp knife, trim any excess dough along the edge of the pie plate and use the tines of a fork to create a decorative edge.

Bake for 50 to 60 minutes, or until the crust starts to brown and the apples are bubbling.

Let cool to room temperature on a wire rack. Cut into slices and serve (and you better save the last slice for me!).

Week-at-a-Glance

TO-DO LIST

Monday

○ _____
○ _____
○ _____
○ _____
○ _____
○ _____
○ _____
○ _____
○ _____

Tuesday

○ _____
○ _____
○ _____
○ _____
○ _____
○ _____
○ _____
○ _____
○ _____

Wednesday

○ _____
○ _____
○ _____
○ _____
○ _____
○ _____
○ _____
○ _____
○ _____

Habit Tracker

HABIT	M	T	W	Th	F	S	Su

What's for Dinner?

M	
T	
W	
Th	
F	
S	
Su	

Thursday

- ◯ _____
- ◯ _____
- ◯ _____
- ◯ _____
- ◯ _____
- ◯ _____
- ◯ _____
- ◯ _____
- ◯ _____

Friday

- ◯ _____
- ◯ _____
- ◯ _____
- ◯ _____
- ◯ _____
- ◯ _____
- ◯ _____
- ◯ _____
- ◯ _____

Saturday

- ◯ _____
- ◯ _____
- ◯ _____
- ◯ _____
- ◯ _____
- ◯ _____
- ◯ _____
- ◯ _____
- ◯ _____

TO-DO LIST

Movement Planner

M	
T	
W	
Th	
F	
S	
Su	

Sunday

- ◯ _____
- ◯ _____
- ◯ _____
- ◯ _____
- ◯ _____
- ◯ _____
- ◯ _____
- ◯ _____
- ◯ _____

TO-DO LIST

Monday

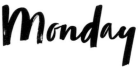

.... / .... / ....

Top Priorities

1. _____
2. _____
3. _____

TO-DOS

- ○ _____
- ○ _____
- ○ _____
- ○ _____
- ○ _____
- ○ _____
- ○ _____
- ○ _____
- ○ _____
- ○ _____

NOTES

MEALS

B	
L	
D	
S	

WATER TRACKER

○ ○ ○ ○ ○ ○ ○ ○ ○

TIME BLOCKING

:	
:	
:	
:	
:	
:	
:	
:	
:	
:	
:	
:	
:	
:	
:	
:	
:	
:	
:	
:	

_____ / _____ / _____

Tuesday

Top Priorities

1. _____
2. _____
3. _____

TO-DOS

- ○ _____
- ○ _____
- ○ _____
- ○ _____
- ○ _____
- ○ _____
- ○ _____
- ○ _____
- ○ _____
- ○ _____
- ○ _____

NOTES

MEALS

B	
L	
D	
S	

WATER TRACKER

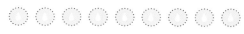

TIME BLOCKING

:	
:	
:	
:	
:	
:	
:	
:	
:	
:	
:	
:	
:	
:	
:	
:	
:	
:	
:	
:	

Wednesday

.... / .... / ....

Top Priorities

1. _____
2. _____
3. _____

TO-DOS

- ○ _____
- ○ _____
- ○ _____
- ○ _____
- ○ _____
- ○ _____
- ○ _____
- ○ _____
- ○ _____
- ○ _____
- ○ _____

NOTES

MEALS

B	
L	
D	
S	

WATER TRACKER

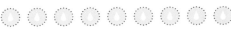

TIME BLOCKING

:	
:	
:	
:	
:	
:	
:	
:	
:	
:	
:	
:	
:	
:	
:	
:	
:	
:	
:	
:	

_____ / _____ / _____

Thursday

Top Priorities

1. _____
2. _____
3. _____

TO-DOS

- ○ _____
- ○ _____
- ○ _____
- ○ _____
- ○ _____
- ○ _____
- ○ _____
- ○ _____
- ○ _____
- ○ _____
- ○ _____

NOTES

MEALS

B	
L	
D	
S	

WATER TRACKER

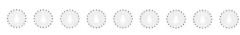

TIME BLOCKING

:	
:	
:	
:	
:	
:	
:	
:	
:	
:	
:	
:	
:	
:	
:	
:	
:	
:	
:	
:	
:	
:	

_____ / _____ / _____

Top Priorities

1. _____
2. _____
3. _____

TO-DOS

○ _____
○ _____
○ _____
○ _____
○ _____
○ _____
○ _____
○ _____
○ _____
○ _____
○ _____

NOTES

MEALS

B	
L	
D	
S	

WATER TRACKER

TIME BLOCKING

:	
:	
:	
:	
:	
:	
:	
:	
:	
:	
:	
:	
:	
:	
:	
:	
:	
:	
:	
:	
:	
:	
:	

_____ / _____ / _____

Saturday & Sunday

Top Priorities

1. _____
2. _____
3. _____

TO-DOS

- ○ _____
- ○ _____
- ○ _____
- ○ _____
- ○ _____
- ○ _____
- ○ _____
- ○ _____
- ○ _____
- ○ _____
- ○ _____

NOTES

MEALS

B	
L	
D	
S	

WATER TRACKER

○ ○ ○ ○ ○ ○ ○ ○ ○

TIME BLOCKING

:	
:	
:	
:	
:	
:	
:	
:	
:	
:	
:	
:	
:	
:	
:	
:	
:	
:	
:	

WEEKLY REFLECTION

How do you feel about what you accomplished in the last seven days?
What went well?

What do you believe to be the obstacles you faced in accomplishing the goals you set last week?

What would a "win" look like for this coming week?

What steps do you need to take to make your "win" a reality?

WEEK 8 ··

Maintaining Motivation

What keeps me motivated?

Do you ever look around and feel like everyone has their life together but you? I can assure you, most people probably don't have it all together. But what many probably do have are systems and routines, a habitual way of living.

Motivation is the idea of accomplishing your goal. Motivation is what gets you started; it's what lights your fire. But motivation is fleeting, and when that feeling leaves you, it's easy to revert to old habits. It's common to want a quick fix in your wellness journey, but there is no fast-forward button. You need to do the work to create permanent change, because when motivation fails, consistency and habits remain.

The first week of any lifestyle change is always the easiest. You feel good, you're amped, you're motivated, you're on a path to a healthier you—you've got that New Year's resolution energy! The second week is more of the same; you're still feeling like you can conquer anything. Come week three, you're getting antsy and want to see changes. You've lost one or two pounds, started writing in your journal, and gotten a few more hours of shut-eye, but it's not enough to get you excited.

And then week four arrives and you're starting to get bored. This is the time to resist the urge for instant gratification and push yourself to make the healthy choice. If you want changes to happen, you must choose this new path and find the inspiration to move forward. Changes will come only from your ability to make a choice other than what you're used to, so consistency can carry you when motivation can't.

COMMUNITY WELLNESS

The pyramid to the right represents a motivational theory proposed by psychologist Abraham Maslow in 1943. Simply referred to as Maslow's hierarchy of needs, it includes five categories that humans need to survive. Not surprisingly, our most basic needs—food, water, warmth, and rest—are the foundation of the pyramid. But did you know that belonging is also essential?

We are not made to exist in isolation. Every single person needs connection and relationships so they can give and receive on a broader scale. The definition of community is a feeling of comradery with others as a result of sharing common attitudes, interests, and goals. I pride myself on helping others form communities that thrive by teaching them how to instill healthier habits through personal coaching. But belonging to something that is greater than ourselves is a common thread we're all trying to weave. I can do HIIT routines for days and eat healthy for weeks on end, but sometimes the only thing that gives me strength is a strong cup of coffee shared with a good friend.

MASLOW'S
hierarchy of needs

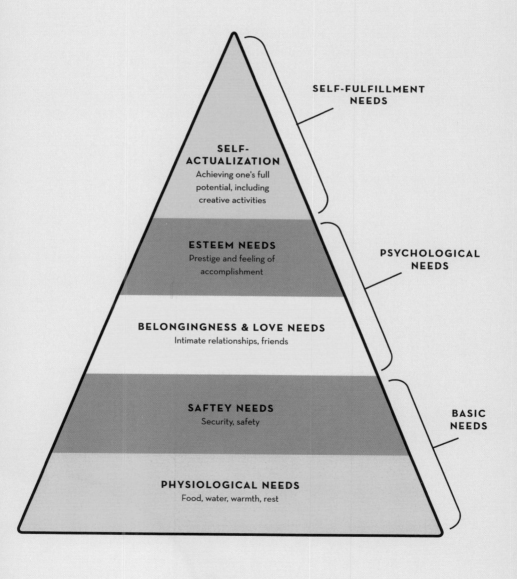

SELF-FULLFILLMENT
NEEDS

**SELF-
ACTUALIZATION**
Achieving one's full
potential, including
creative activities

ESTEEM NEEDS
Prestige and feeling of
accomplishment

PSYCHOLOGICAL
NEEDS

BELONGINGNESS & LOVE NEEDS
Intimate relationships, friends

SAFTEY NEEDS
Security, safety

BASIC
NEEDS

PHYSIOLOGICAL NEEDS
Food, water, warmth, rest

What is your reason for embarking on this journey to a healthier life-style?

_____

_____

_____

List three people who inspire you. What are the qualities they possess that you find most inspirational?

_____

_____

Now, what do you have in common with these people?

_____

_____

_____

Define your why. Really think about why you want to live a healthier lifestyle. Is it to set an example for your children? Is it to feel better in your skin? Write your reasoning down and look back at it on days when you're feeling unmotivated.

_____

_____

_____

_____

THE POWER OF COMMUNITY EXERCISE

One way to interact with your community is through movement and exercise. If you're lacking motivation to get moving, it's okay. You are not alone. Exercising by yourself can seem like a chore, especially if it has been a while since your last squat or plank. My recommendation is to find a virtual fitness class or a group in your community or even one dedicated friend to sweat with. This can provide just the boost you need to get going!

Here are a few reasons why:

Accountability. It's really easy to slack off when you are working out on your own. Group workouts can encourage accountability and help you keep your eye on the prize. Group challenges are also a great way to keep motivated. Try creating a step-count goal with some friends. There are plenty of apps that can help you keep track!

Change of pace. Instead of the usual drinks-and-dinner outing with your friend group, switch it up! Group exercise classes, whether virtual or in person, can be entertaining and take some of the seriousness out of a traditional workout or gym visit. Take it up a notch with a theme! Coordinate outfits and exercises with your favorite TV show, genre of music, or pop culture era.

Effective movement. Have you ever wondered, *Am I doing this right?* Take the guesswork out of exercising and get coached by a human! Coaches can ensure that your workouts are safe and effective for the entire group.

Positive lifestyle change. Incorporating a group of supportive friends into your fitness journey can make a long-lasting difference. It is proven that a positive support group can reduce stress and discourage unhealthy habits.[7] They can motivate you and help you maintain all the habits you are adding into your life.

GRACE AND THE VILLAGE

When my two girls were little, we lived in a townhouse in Alexandria, Virginia. It was the perfect size—big enough for hosting parties and gatherings but small enough to feel cozy, safe, and low maintenance.

On September 11, 2013, at two o'clock in the morning, we were woken up by the dog barking incessantly at the windows. "Shut up, Grace!" I yelled from my melatonin-induced slumber. Grace continued to bark. I could no longer ignore the ongoing annoyance, so I got up and stumbled to the window. I was completely shocked to see fire engines, lights blazing, and smoke coming from the house right next door. Grace was trying to alert us.

At the very moment I yelled to my husband that the house was on fire, there was a loud bang on our door—the fire department. He ran to the door, I ran to the kids, and in a blur, we all exited the house and piled into the car. Did I mention it was 2:00 a.m.?

Once we got the all clear from the fire department, we headed to my mom's house. Three of the townhomes, ours included, had suffered smoke, water, and fire damage, which left us displaced for two months. Thankfully, no one was injured, and we were able to stay with my mom for a few weeks.

We had a full house, including my mom, my sister-in-law, my cousin, me, my husband, the two girls, and of course, Grace Ball (Grace's middle name)! It was one big happy family. The days were filled with meal prep, laughter, crying, all the emotions—and it was wonderful.

This was the beginning of growing our village. We sold our townhouse, my mom's house, and two rental properties, and we purchased our first multigenerational home with my mom, cousin, kids, and Grace. Turns out we were living that Blue Zone life (see page 98) before we even knew what it was.

Since then, my cousin and sister-in-law have moved on to their own lives, and we've added two boys, a nanny who is like family, and another goldendoodle. There is something special about my children being able to grow up in the same house as their grandma. There is never a dull moment, ever. And I can, without a doubt, say that my husband and I would not be able to live the life we live without our village.

Practice

Off the top of my head, I can think of three people I could call at any given moment for help with anything. We all need that security. In this next section, you will begin to build out your support system. Relationships are something that you have to actively maintain. If you don't, they will eventually brown out and wither away. So, let's water those relationships!

Connect with a person or group who motivates you to make healthier choices. This may involve finding a running or walking group, joining a local community center, or maybe exchanging recipes with your neighbor. We all need a little external motivation sometimes!

Who is in your village? This can be like-minded neighbors or someone at your children's school, but whoever they are, they should be people you could call for any reason.

When something good happens, who is the first person you want to call? Why?

_____

_____

_____

_____

_____

_____

_____

_____

Connection is important. Call someone in your village just to say hello. Who is that person?

_____

_____

_____

_____

_____

_____

_____

_____

Week-at-a-Glance

TO-DO LIST

Monday

- ◯ _____
- ◯ _____
- ◯ _____
- ◯ _____
- ◯ _____
- ◯ _____
- ◯ _____
- ◯ _____
- ◯ _____

Tuesday

- ◯ _____
- ◯ _____
- ◯ _____
- ◯ _____
- ◯ _____
- ◯ _____
- ◯ _____
- ◯ _____
- ◯ _____

Wednesday

- ◯ _____
- ◯ _____
- ◯ _____
- ◯ _____
- ◯ _____
- ◯ _____
- ◯ _____
- ◯ _____
- ◯ _____

Habit Tracker

HABIT	M	T	W	Th	F	S	Su

What's for Dinner?

M	
T	
W	
Th	
F	
S	
Su	

___ / ___ / ___   ___ — ___ / ___ / ___

Thursday

- ○ _____
- ○ _____
- ○ _____
- ○ _____
- ○ _____
- ○ _____
- ○ _____
- ○ _____
- ○ _____

Friday

- ○ _____
- ○ _____
- ○ _____
- ○ _____
- ○ _____
- ○ _____
- ○ _____
- ○ _____
- ○ _____

Saturday

- ○ _____
- ○ _____
- ○ _____
- ○ _____
- ○ _____
- ○ _____
- ○ _____
- ○ _____
- ○ _____

Movement Planner

M	
T	
W	
Th	
F	
S	
Su	

Sunday

- ○ _____
- ○ _____
- ○ _____
- ○ _____
- ○ _____
- ○ _____
- ○ _____
- ○ _____
- ○ _____

Monday

.... / .... / ....

Top Priorities

1. _____
2. _____
3. _____

TO-DOS

- ○ _____
- ○ _____
- ○ _____
- ○ _____
- ○ _____
- ○ _____
- ○ _____
- ○ _____
- ○ _____
- ○ _____
- ○ _____

NOTES

MEALS

B	
L	
D	
S	

WATER TRACKER

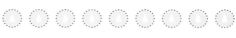

TIME BLOCKING

:	
:	
:	
:	
:	
:	
:	
:	
:	
:	
:	
:	
:	
:	
:	
:	
:	
:	
:	
:	
:	
:	

_____ / _____ / _____

Tuesday

Top Priorities

1. _____
2. _____
3. _____

TO-DOS

- ○ _____
- ○ _____
- ○ _____
- ○ _____
- ○ _____
- ○ _____
- ○ _____
- ○ _____
- ○ _____
- ○ _____
- ○ _____

NOTES

MEALS

B	
L	
D	
S	

WATER TRACKER

TIME BLOCKING

:	
:	
:	
:	
:	
:	
:	
:	
:	
:	
:	
:	
:	
:	
:	
:	
:	
:	
:	

Wednesday

_____ / _____ / _____

Top Priorities

1. _____
2. _____
3. _____

TO-DOS

○ _____
○ _____
○ _____
○ _____
○ _____
○ _____
○ _____
○ _____
○ _____
○ _____
○ _____

NOTES

MEALS

B	
L	
D	
S	

WATER TRACKER

○ ○ ○ ○ ○ ○ ○ ○ ○

TIME BLOCKING

:
:
:
:
:
:
:
:
:
:
:
:
:
:
:
:
:
:
:
:
:

_____ / _____ / _____

Thursday

Top Priorities

1. _____
2. _____
3. _____

TO-DOS

- ○ _____
- ○ _____
- ○ _____
- ○ _____
- ○ _____
- ○ _____
- ○ _____
- ○ _____
- ○ _____
- ○ _____
- ○ _____

NOTES

MEALS

B	
L	
D	
S	

WATER TRACKER

TIME BLOCKING

:	
:	
:	
:	
:	
:	
:	
:	
:	
:	
:	
:	
:	
:	
:	
:	
:	
:	
:	
:	
:	

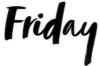

.... / .... / ....

Top Priorities

1. _____

2. _____

3. _____

TO-DOS

- ○ _____
- ○ _____
- ○ _____
- ○ _____
- ○ _____
- ○ _____
- ○ _____
- ○ _____
- ○ _____
- ○ _____
- ○ _____

NOTES

MEALS

B	
L	
D	
S	

WATER TRACKER

TIME BLOCKING

:	
:	
:	
:	
:	
:	
:	
:	
:	
:	
:	
:	
:	
:	
:	
:	
:	
:	
:	
:	

.... / .... / ....

Saturday & Sunday

Top Priorities

1. _____

2. _____

3. _____

MEALS

B	
L	
D	
S	

WATER TRACKER

◯ ◯ ◯ ◯ ◯ ◯ ◯ ◯ ◯

TO-DOS

- ◯ _____
- ◯ _____
- ◯ _____
- ◯ _____
- ◯ _____
- ◯ _____
- ◯ _____
- ◯ _____
- ◯ _____
- ◯ _____
- ◯ _____

TIME BLOCKING

:	
:	
:	
:	
:	
:	
:	
:	
:	
:	
:	
:	
:	
:	
:	
:	
:	
:	
:	
:	
:	

NOTES

WEEKLY REFLECTION

How do you feel about what you accomplished in the last seven days? What went well?

What do you believe to be the obstacles you faced in accomplishing the goals you set last week?

What would a "win" look like for this coming week?

What steps do you need to take to make your "win" a reality?

"You don't have to be positive all the time. It's perfectly OK to feel sad, angry, annoyed, frustrated, scared and anxious. Having feelings doesn't make you a negative person. It makes you human."

—LORI DESCHENE

Mental Wellness

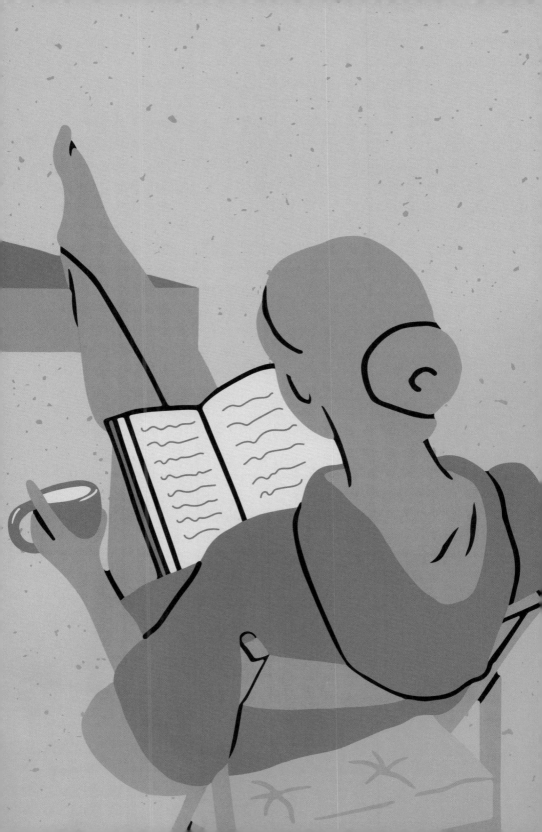

WEEK 9 ·······································

Gratitude

We have spent a lot of time addressing the needs of the physical body. Now let's work on mindset, as it plays a significant role in how we approach the other aspects of our lives. It's easier to focus on what we don't have than what we do, so we have to work extra hard to intentionally maintain a positive mindset. That means we have to figure out a way to integrate gratitude into our daily life.

 gratitude: *the quality of being thankful or appreciative*

Many therapists feel that practicing gratitude can have a significant positive influence on our physical and mental health. In fact, it's supported by research and anecdotal evidence that journaling gratitude on a regular basis is a powerful habit to create when it comes to developing a positive mindset.[8]

However, much like any other healthy habit, practicing it with consistency can often be difficult, even though we know it's good for us. I like to start every day with gratitude. I am often overscheduled and overstressed, so as part of my morning routine, I write down three things that I am grateful for in my journal.

4 REASONS TO
Start Journaling

REASON 1:
LET IT ALL OUT

The mind is a powerful thing that can make problems seem larger than they actually are. Journaling is a good way to let it all out and maintain perspective.

REASON 2:
SPEAK OPENLY

Your journal is your safe space. You can speak openly about your thoughts, fears, and ideas without judgement.

REASON 3:
STAY MENTALLY ACTIVE

The mind needs activity just like the body. Journaling is a good way to stay mentally active while utilizing a healthy outlet.

REASON 4:
CULTIVATE GRATITUDE

With journaling, you can not only write what's bothering you, but you can remember all you have to be grateful for. Practicing gratitude is a great way to remain grounded.

DON'T BREAK THE CHAIN

Like exercise and healthy eating, journaling needs to be done consistently in order to deliver the benefits. I have been a health and wellness coach for years and believe me, I have heard every excuse in the book. In fact, I've probably used every excuse in the book myself. Creating new habits, such as practicing gratitude or journaling consistently, are not immune to those excuses. If you feel like you "don't have time" or think, I've tried it, I just can't keep it up, *think again*. You may have to work at it, but you can do it. Eventually, your new habits will begin to feel second nature, and you'll reap the benefits in the form of better sleep, hydration, and a positive outlook on life.

Comedian Jerry Seinfeld gave a young comic named Brad Isaac some advice about how to write and create material. Keep a calendar, he told him, and mark each day that you write jokes with an X. Seeing all those X's will motivate you to keep the habit chain going—your job is simply to not break the chain.

Success is a matter of momentum and consistency. Once you get something going and keep at it, keeping it moving in the right direction will start to become easier. Begin with one day, then another, then another, and don't break the chain.

Practice

Set aside 10 minutes each morning or evening to journal and practice gratitude. Need some guidance? Use the prompts on the opposite page to get you going.

If you need more inspiration, I've included 30 days of journal prompts in the Resources section (see page 226).

What am I already grateful for in my life?

_____

_____

_____

_____

_____

_____

_____

How can I incorporate gratitude into my daily life? (Remember, I committed to spending 5 minutes each day writing down the things I'm grateful for, which has worked for me.)

_____

_____

_____

_____

_____

Who makes you smile? Why?

_____

_____

_____

_____

Week-at-a-Glance

TO-DO LIST

Monday

- ◯ ....
- ◯ ....
- ◯ ....
- ◯ ....
- ◯ ....
- ◯ ....
- ◯ ....
- ◯ ....
- ◯ ....

Tuesday

- ◯ ....
- ◯ ....
- ◯ ....
- ◯ ....
- ◯ ....
- ◯ ....
- ◯ ....
- ◯ ....
- ◯ ....

Wednesday

- ◯ ....
- ◯ ....
- ◯ ....
- ◯ ....
- ◯ ....
- ◯ ....
- ◯ ....
- ◯ ....
- ◯ ....

Habit Tracker

HABIT	M	T	W	Th	F	S	Su

What's for Dinner?

M	
T	
W	
Th	
F	
S	
Su	

Thursday

○ _____
○ _____
○ _____
○ _____
○ _____
○ _____
○ _____
○ _____
○ _____

Friday

○ _____
○ _____
○ _____
○ _____
○ _____
○ _____
○ _____
○ _____
○ _____

Saturday

○ _____
○ _____
○ _____
○ _____
○ _____
○ _____
○ _____
○ _____
○ _____

TO-DO LIST

Movement Planner

M	
T	
W	
Th	
F	
S	
Su	

Sunday

○ _____
○ _____
○ _____
○ _____
○ _____
○ _____
○ _____
○ _____
○ _____

TO-DO LIST

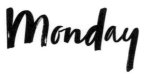

Monday

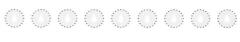

Top Priorities

1. _____
2. _____
3. _____

TO-DOS

- ○ _____
- ○ _____
- ○ _____
- ○ _____
- ○ _____
- ○ _____
- ○ _____
- ○ _____
- ○ _____
- ○ _____
- ○ _____

NOTES

MEALS

B	
L	
D	
S	

WATER TRACKER

○ ○ ○ ○ ○ ○ ○ ○ ○

TIME BLOCKING

:	
:	
:	
:	
:	
:	
:	
:	
:	
:	
:	
:	
:	
:	
:	
:	
:	
:	
:	
:	
:	

_____ / _____ / _____

Tuesday

Top Priorities

1. _____
2. _____
3. _____

MEALS

B	
L	
D	
S	

WATER TRACKER

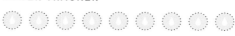

TO-DOS

- ○ _____
- ○ _____
- ○ _____
- ○ _____
- ○ _____
- ○ _____
- ○ _____
- ○ _____
- ○ _____
- ○ _____
- ○ _____

TIME BLOCKING

:	
:	
:	
:	
:	
:	
:	
:	
:	
:	
:	
:	
:	
:	
:	
:	
:	
:	
:	
:	
:	

NOTES

Wednesday

_____ / _____ / _____

Top Priorities

1. _____
2. _____
3. _____

MEALS

B	
L	
D	
S	

WATER TRACKER

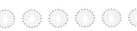

TO-DOS

- ○ _____
- ○ _____
- ○ _____
- ○ _____
- ○ _____
- ○ _____
- ○ _____
- ○ _____
- ○ _____
- ○ _____
- ○ _____

TIME BLOCKING

:	
:	
:	
:	
:	
:	
:	
:	
:	
:	
:	
:	
:	
:	
:	
:	
:	
:	
:	

NOTES

_____ / _____ / _____

Thursday

Top Priorities

1. _____
2. _____
3. _____

MEALS

B	
L	
D	
S	

WATER TRACKER

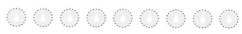

TO-DOS

- ○ _____
- ○ _____
- ○ _____
- ○ _____
- ○ _____
- ○ _____
- ○ _____
- ○ _____
- ○ _____
- ○ _____
- ○ _____

TIME BLOCKING

:	
:	
:	
:	
:	
:	
:	
:	
:	
:	
:	
:	
:	
:	
:	
:	
:	
:	
:	
:	

NOTES

Friday

.... / .... / ....

Top Priorities

1. _____
2. _____
3. _____

TO-DOS

○ _____
○ _____
○ _____
○ _____
○ _____
○ _____
○ _____
○ _____
○ _____
○ _____
○ _____
○ _____

NOTES

MEALS

B	
L	
D	
S	

WATER TRACKER

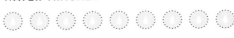

TIME BLOCKING

:	
:	
:	
:	
:	
:	
:	
:	
:	
:	
:	
:	
:	
:	
:	
:	
:	
:	
:	

_____ / _____ / _____

Saturday & Sunday

Top Priorities

1. _____
2. _____
3. _____

TO-DOS

- ○ _____
- ○ _____
- ○ _____
- ○ _____
- ○ _____
- ○ _____
- ○ _____
- ○ _____
- ○ _____
- ○ _____
- ○ _____

NOTES

MEALS

B	
L	
D	
S	

WATER TRACKER

TIME BLOCKING

:	
:	
:	
:	
:	
:	
:	
:	
:	
:	
:	
:	
:	
:	
:	
:	
:	
:	
:	
:	
:	
:	

WEEKLY REFLECTION

How do you feel about what you accomplished in the last seven days? What went well?

What do you believe to be the obstacles you faced in accomplishing the goals you set last week?

What would a "win" look like for this coming week?

What steps do you need to take to make your "win" a reality?

WEEK 10 ···

Slowing Down

In a world that often seems fast-paced and overconnected, it is easy to get swept up in the feeling of needing to do more just to keep up.

The problem is that we spend so much energy and mental capacity trying to fit it all in that we can't enjoy the life that is happening all around us. That frantic, overwhelmed feeling you get is your body telling you to slow down!

If you don't make time to slow down and enjoy the books or the knitting, you will become an overscheduled, overstressed ball of tension. Believe me, nobody wants that.

Reacting to stress is a normal adaptive response, but too much of it can eventually lead to disease.[9] If you have poor coping strategies, this can happen precipitously. Today, where virtual reality makes everything accessible, it's important to take a minute, or ten, to step back, slow down, and just breathe! Try deleting social media from your phone on the weekends or setting hard boundaries around work emails. When you intentionally slow down, it helps you become more present and mindful in your days and, in turn, more intentional and less reactive to the stressors in your life.

WAYS TO SLOW DOWN & DECREASE STRESS

Get out in nature

Several studies show that nature walks improve the memory in ways that other types of walks don't.[10] Additionally, anxiety, depression, and other mental health issues may all be eased by spending some time in nature—especially when that's combined with exercise.[11]

Start your days slower

If you find yourself constantly feeling rushed in the mornings, try waking up 15 minutes earlier. This will allow you to take your mornings slower and help you carry that feeling throughout the rest of the day. And don't forget to set a realistic morning routine and follow it, which will keep you from trying to do more than time allows.

Try square breathing

This is a deep breathing technique that is often used with children to help them deal with big feelings, but it works great for adults too because it forces you to slow down, which will lower your stress. Try these simple steps as you read:

1. Slowly exhale until your lungs are empty.
2. Then slowly inhale to the count of four.
3. Hold your breath for another slow count of four.
4. Exhale through your mouth for the same slow count of four, expelling all the air from your lungs and abdomen. Be conscious of the feeling of the air leaving your lungs.
5. Hold your breath for the same slow count of four before repeating this process once.

The Mayo Clinic has stated that deep breathing can calm and regulate the nervous system.[12]

Find a hobby!

Take up a new hobby and do it at least once a week. This can be anything you enjoy and that makes you happy. (According to my husband, shopping is not a good hobby for me.) My go-tos are a nice Mosaic puzzle or baking for my neighbors.

STRESS MANAGEMENT

While too much stress can have a negative effect on your body, stress itself is not necessarily a bad thing. It's your body's way of letting you know something is not as it should be. The goal is not to completely eliminate stress but to figure out ways to manage and cope with it.

Your mindset matters. Try changing your thought patterns about what's causing you stress. Be mindful of where your thoughts are taking you. There will always be stressors in life and while you can't control when they appear, you can learn to recognize and control how you respond to those stressors.

"Each person deserves a day away in which no problems are confronted, no solutions are searched for."
- Maya Angelou

MANAGING YOUR STRESS LEVELS

As I mentioned, stressors are everywhere. Rather than replaying your stressful moments over in your head, talk or write about them and move on. Avoid revisiting these moments once you've expressed everything on paper or verbally. Research shows that those who talk about stressful situations release hormones that reduce negative feelings associated with those stressors.[13] Problems often seem larger than life in our minds, but once we address them head-on and develop a plan to fix them, we notice a sudden release. That's our stress floating away!

Proper planning is also a really good tool for reducing stress. Prioritize your to-dos and focus on the low-hanging fruit, such as responding to simple emails or handling schedule conflicts, first. This will quickly free up mental capacity to focus on larger tasks. In times when you are really overwhelmed, go back to the basics,

What do you do when you're stressed out or up against a wall?

_____

_____

_____

_____

_____

_____

_____

_____

Do you feel that your stress response is a healthy one? If not, how can you change it? If it is, brainstorm other tools that can help you manage stress.

_____

_____

_____

_____

_____

_____

_____

_____

and lean into what you can control. If your children are sick, you may lose your workouts and fall behind on work tasks, but you can control your hydration (Week 4) and sleep hygiene (Week 2).

When all else fails, a good dose of perspective can go a long way. Think about your stressor in terms of longevity. Will who did (or didn't) do the dishes matter in one week? How about one month or even one year? It's important to think about things in a broader, more objective context. It's hard to see the forest for the trees, so take a step back and regain that view!

Practice

Set aside 5 minutes every day this week to do the body scan on the following page. Then jot down your stress level in the Notes section of the Week-at-a-Glance page.

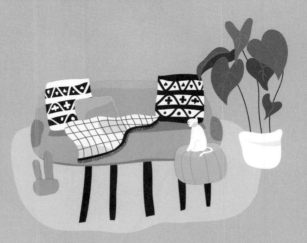

BODY SCAN
exercise

1. Set a 5-minute timer and perform the following actions until the time is up.

2. Sit or lie down in a quiet place with no distractions.

3. Starting at the top of your head and slowly going down to your toes, become aware of all of your physical sensations. Notice the smells, the sounds around you. Is your breathing deep or shallow? Are you noticing any tension? If so, simply acknowledge it and continue to scan your body. Observe only—no judgment.

4. If your mind starts to wander, focus on where you are on your body and continue to scan.

5. Take mental note of what you are feeling physically. Does your jaw feel tight? Are your fists clenched? Are you able to just fall and sink into the floor?

6. Take mental note of what you are feeling emotionally. Are you having a hard time keeping your mind from wandering? Do you feel anxious? Curious about the time?

7. Take mental note of your thoughts.

Based on this scan, what have you learned about yourself?

_____

_____

_____

_____

_____

_____

_____

_____

_____

_____

_____

_____

_____

_____

_____

_____

_____

_____

_____

_____

Week-at-a-Glance

TO-DO LIST

Monday

- ◯ _____
- ◯ _____
- ◯ _____
- ◯ _____
- ◯ _____
- ◯ _____
- ◯ _____
- ◯ _____
- ◯ _____

Tuesday

- ◯ _____
- ◯ _____
- ◯ _____
- ◯ _____
- ◯ _____
- ◯ _____
- ◯ _____
- ◯ _____
- ◯ _____

Wednesday

- ◯ _____
- ◯ _____
- ◯ _____
- ◯ _____
- ◯ _____
- ◯ _____
- ◯ _____
- ◯ _____
- ◯ _____

Habit Tracker

HABIT	M	T	W	Th	F	S	Su

What's for Dinner?

M	
T	
W	
Th	
F	
S	
Su	

Thursday

- ◯ _____
- ◯ _____
- ◯ _____
- ◯ _____
- ◯ _____
- ◯ _____
- ◯ _____
- ◯ _____
- ◯ _____

Friday

- ◯ _____
- ◯ _____
- ◯ _____
- ◯ _____
- ◯ _____
- ◯ _____
- ◯ _____
- ◯ _____
- ◯ _____

Saturday

- ◯ _____
- ◯ _____
- ◯ _____
- ◯ _____
- ◯ _____
- ◯ _____
- ◯ _____
- ◯ _____
- ◯ _____

TO-DO LIST

Movement Planner

M	
T	
W	
Th	
F	
S	
Su	

Sunday

- ◯ _____
- ◯ _____
- ◯ _____
- ◯ _____
- ◯ _____
- ◯ _____
- ◯ _____
- ◯ _____
- ◯ _____

TO-DO LIST

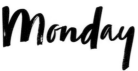

Monday

_____ / _____ / _____

Top Priorities

1. _____
2. _____
3. _____

TO-DOS

- ○ _____
- ○ _____
- ○ _____
- ○ _____
- ○ _____
- ○ _____
- ○ _____
- ○ _____
- ○ _____
- ○ _____
- ○ _____

NOTES

MEALS

B	
L	
D	
S	

WATER TRACKER

○ ○ ○ ○ ○ ○ ○ ○ ○

TIME BLOCKING

:	
:	
:	
:	
:	
:	
:	
:	
:	
:	
:	
:	
:	
:	
:	
:	
:	
:	
:	
:	
:	
:	

_____ / _____ / _____

Tuesday

Top Priorities

1. _____
2. _____
3. _____

TO-DOS

- ○ _____
- ○ _____
- ○ _____
- ○ _____
- ○ _____
- ○ _____
- ○ _____
- ○ _____
- ○ _____
- ○ _____
- ○ _____

NOTES

MEALS

B	
L	
D	
S	

WATER TRACKER

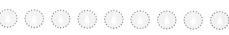

TIME BLOCKING

:	
:	
:	
:	
:	
:	
:	
:	
:	
:	
:	
:	
:	
:	
:	
:	
:	
:	
:	
:	

Wednesday

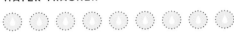 / /

Top Priorities

1. _____
2. _____
3. _____

TO-DOS

- ○ _____
- ○ _____
- ○ _____
- ○ _____
- ○ _____
- ○ _____
- ○ _____
- ○ _____
- ○ _____
- ○ _____
- ○ _____

NOTES

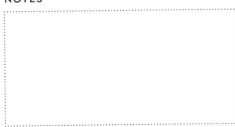

MEALS

B	
L	
D	
S	

WATER TRACKER

○ ○ ○ ○ ○ ○ ○ ○ ○

TIME BLOCKING

:	
:	
:	
:	
:	
:	
:	
:	
:	
:	
:	
:	
:	
:	
:	
:	
:	
:	
:	
:	
:	
:	

Thursday

_____ / _____ / _____

Top Priorities

1. _____
2. _____
3. _____

TO-DOS

- ○ _____
- ○ _____
- ○ _____
- ○ _____
- ○ _____
- ○ _____
- ○ _____
- ○ _____
- ○ _____
- ○ _____
- ○ _____

NOTES

MEALS

B	
L	
D	
S	

WATER TRACKER

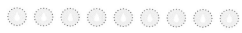

TIME BLOCKING

:	
:	
:	
:	
:	
:	
:	
:	
:	
:	
:	
:	
:	
:	
:	
:	
:	
:	
:	
:	
:	

Friday

.... / ...... / ....

Top Priorities

1. _____

2. _____

3. _____

TO-DOS

- ○ _____
- ○ _____
- ○ _____
- ○ _____
- ○ _____
- ○ _____
- ○ _____
- ○ _____
- ○ _____
- ○ _____
- ○ _____

NOTES

MEALS

B	
L	
D	
S	

WATER TRACKER

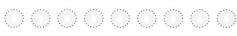

TIME BLOCKING

:	
:	
:	
:	
:	
:	
:	
:	
:	
:	
:	
:	
:	
:	
:	
:	
:	
:	
:	
:	
:	

_____ / _____ / _____

Saturday & Sunday

Top Priorities

1. _____
2. _____
3. _____

TO-DOS

○ _____
○ _____
○ _____
○ _____
○ _____
○ _____
○ _____
○ _____
○ _____
○ _____
○ _____

NOTES

MEALS

B	
L	
D	
S	

WATER TRACKER

○ ○ ○ ○ ○ ○ ○ ○ ○

TIME BLOCKING

:	
:	
:	
:	
:	
:	
:	
:	
:	
:	
:	
:	
:	
:	
:	
:	
:	
:	

WEEKLY REFLECTION

How do you feel about what you accomplished in the last seven days? What went well?

What do you believe to be the obstacles you faced in accomplishing the goals you set last week?

What would a "win" look like for this coming week?

What steps do you need to take to make your "win" a reality?

"If you look at what you have in life, you'll always have more. If you look at what you don't have in life, you'll never have enough."

— OPRAH WINFREY

Financial Wellness

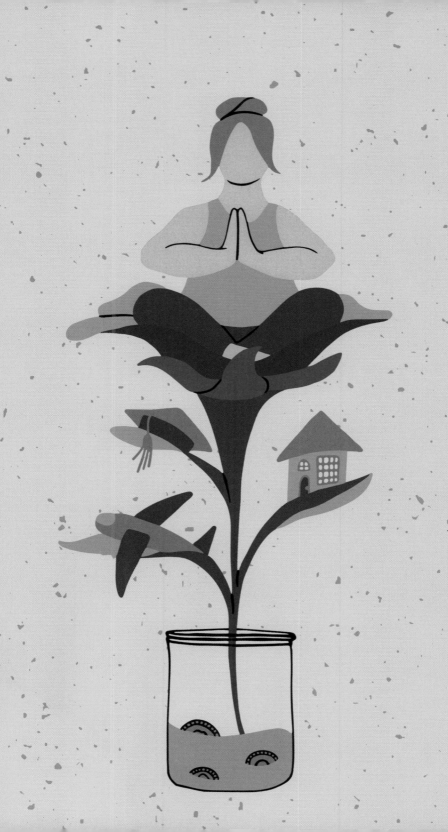

WEEK 11 ··

Financial Knowledge

Financial knowledge gives you power. No matter how much money you have, knowing how the financial world works and what you can do to start growing your finances will lead you to a lifestyle where you have options. Keeping track of how much money you're bringing in and having a plan for how you are going to use that money will lower your stress and let you focus on other things.

As with managing any kind of stress, learning to spend intentionally and not impulsively will take you to the next level. While I'm not qualified to offer financial advice, I can recommend tools to get comfortable looking at and thinking about your money differently.

Here are a few key financial terms and their definitions that may be helpful to know along the way:

Compounding interest. The interest you earn on interest, usually resulting from money you have previously saved or invested.

Investment. Something you spend your money on that will return financial gain.

Money plan. A less polarizing term for a *budget*. It is a plan for every dollar that comes into your household, including spending and saving and eventually investing or donating.

Spending trigger. An event that happens to get you to spend money. Example: You're out and hungry, so you stop by a restaurant and grab a bite to eat.

TIME / VALUE / MONEY

There is one thing you have that has more value than money and that's your time. It's something you cannot get back once it's spent. You can always make more money, but once those hours, days, and years are gone, sadly, there is no returning. That makes your ability to control how you spend your time the ultimate goal. If you, like most people, wake up, go to work, spend eight hours doing a job you really don't like, go home, do chores around the house, eat, rinse, repeat, then your time is being dictated by your job, or your boss.

Read that again. How you spend your time is controlled by something or someone else.

Now I want you to imagine that you have complete control over how you spend your days. Money is no object.

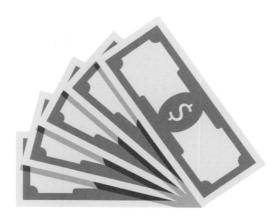

What would your ideal day look like? Describe it below.

_____

_____

_____

_____

_____

_____

_____

_____

What steps can you take to start making your ideal day a reality?

_____

_____

_____

_____

_____

Create one goal that will bring you closer to your ideal life. Here's an example: I want to secure a new job in the next six months that allows me to work from home.

_____

_____

_____

COMPOUNDING INTEREST 101

Okay, stay with me, as I can already sense your eyes glazing over. Compounding interest isn't the sexiest topic, but I actually think you'll enjoy this quick lesson. Simply speaking, compounding interest is the interest you earn on your interest; that is, your money is making money or passive income. Why should you spend your valuable time making money? Put those dollars to work!

An easy math equation:

- **Year 1,** you save $100 at 5% interest compounded annually. By the end of the year, you have $105.

- **Year 2,** you earn 5% interest on that $105. By the end of the year, you will have $110.25.

- **Year 3,** you earn 5% interest on $110.15. By the end of the year, you will have $115.76.
  You can see where this is going.

Now add a few zeros to that number.

- **$10,000** turns into $11,576.00.

- **$100,000** turns into $115,760.00

- **$1,000,000** turns into $1,115,760.00

Now, let's invest and compound more frequently to really see the power!

- **Year 1,** you save $500 a month at 7% interest compounded monthly. By the end of the year, you have $6,732.44.

- **Year 2,** you continue to save $500 a month and you earn 7% interest on that $6,732.44. By the end of the year, you will have $13,415.42.

Stick to the plan, and by year 10 you will have accumulated $87,547.23.

The best part is you don't have do anything! Compounding interest means that your money is doing the work. All you have to do is save it and not touch it! This is where investing in the stock markets and your 401K come into play.

Your turn.

Do you have a 401K or an IRA? If so, how much do you contribute each month? If not, start one. Any amount is better than nothing.

Does your employer match your contributions?

Do you have an understanding of basic investing? If not, spend 15 minutes to research online!

How did my husband and I explain compounding interest to four kids ranging in age from three to thirteen, you ask? We used chocolate chips of course! We gave each child a choice. They could choose 10 chocolate chips right now, but they wouldn't get any more for the next 5 minutes or they could choose 1 chocolate chip, compounded at 100% interest every minute for 5 minutes.

Two children chose 10 chocolate chips up front. The other two children chose 1 chocolate chip, compounded at 100% interest for 5 minutes. On every minute, we doubled the number of chocolate chips for the kids who chose 100% compounded interest. The other two sat and watched their 10 chips sit unchanged.

By the end of 5 minutes, two children had 10 chocolate chips and two had 32 chocolate chips.

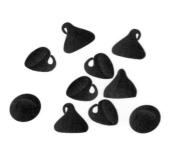

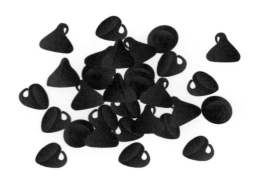

10 CHOCOLATE CHIPS   32 CHOCOLATE CHIPS

It was an easy exercise to explain why, as long as you don't touch it, investing makes more sense than just saving your money.

COMPLETE YOUR FINANCIAL REPORT CARD

Use these next few pages to keep track of your day-to-day spending habits and analyze your feelings about your current finances. Start by writing down how you spend for three days using the Finance Tracking pages. If you need more, you can find a link to the spreadsheet on my website (see Resources, page 228) and print out as many pages as you need.

DATE	EXPENSE	AMOUNT	PAYMENT METHOD	FEELINGS	MERCHANT
03/01	Groceries	$134.82	Debit Card	Great, I was able to prep for the week	Whole Foods
03/02	Coffee	$4.72	Credit Card	In a rush, just wanted coffee	Starbucks
03/02	Lunch	$15.76	Credit Card	Work lunch with coworker	La Brea Café

Practice

This week, complete Your Financial Report Card. What are your spending triggers? Do you browse Amazon at night when you're bored? Do you window-shop when you're sad? I'm a stress shopper. If I'm stressed, I browse Saks online, put a bunch of stuff in my cart, and then shut the browser. By understanding your intentions behind what you spend your money on, you can then evaluate how to change or strengthen your relationship with your finances.

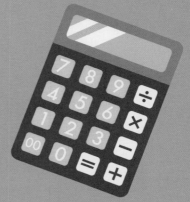

YOUR FINANCIAL
report card

DATE	EXPENSE	AMOUNT	PAYMENT METHO

FEELINGS	MERCHANT

YOUR FINANCIAL
report card

DATE	EXPENSE	AMOUNT	PAYMENT METHO

FEELINGS	MERCHANT

YOUR FINANCIAL
report card

DATE	EXPENSE	AMOUNT	PAYMENT METHO

FEELINGS	MERCHANT

You tracked your spending. Now what? Work on flexing your financial muscles, of course. Identify three things:

What excites you about your spending? (Example: I was able to stick to my spending plan at Target!)

_____

_____

_____

_____

_____

What surprises you about your spending? (Example: I shop online at night when I'm bored. Amazon makes consumerism way too easy! Amirite?)

_____

_____

_____

_____

_____

_____

What concerns you about your spending? (Example: I used DoorDash three times in five days. Oh my!)

_____

_____

_____

_____

_____

_____

_____

_____

_____

_____

Now that you've evaluated your spending habits, set three financial goals. Be SMART (Specific, Measurable, Attainable, Relevant, and Time-Bound) with your goals. (For example, I want to save $1,000 in the next 6 months.)

_____

_____

_____

_____

_____

_____

Define what success means to you. Does having a powerful, high-profile job and lifestyle mean success, or is success being a stay-at-home parent? Maybe a combination of the two? There is no wrong answer. At the end of your life, you will have been successful if . . .

_____

_____

_____

_____

_____

_____

_____

_____

_____

What do you spend money on that you can cut back on? Be honest!

_____

_____

_____

_____

_____

Do you have an emergency fund or at least three months of living expenses in a savings account? If not, how would you sustain yourself in the event of a job loss or medical emergency?

_____

_____

_____

_____

_____

_____

_____

Do you consider yourself financially knowledgeable? If not, why? If yes, what is one aspect of money you want to learn more about?

_____

_____

_____

_____

_____

_____

_____

_____

Week-at-a-Glance

TO-DO LIST

Monday

- ○ _____
- ○ _____
- ○ _____
- ○ _____
- ○ _____
- ○ _____
- ○ _____
- ○ _____
- ○ _____

Tuesday

- ○ _____
- ○ _____
- ○ _____
- ○ _____
- ○ _____
- ○ _____
- ○ _____
- ○ _____
- ○ _____

Wednesday

- ○ _____
- ○ _____
- ○ _____
- ○ _____
- ○ _____
- ○ _____
- ○ _____
- ○ _____
- ○ _____

Habit Tracker

HABIT	M	T	W	Th	F	S	Su

What's for Dinner?

M	
T	
W	
Th	
F	
S	
Su	

Thursday

- ◯ _____
- ◯ _____
- ◯ _____
- ◯ _____
- ◯ _____
- ◯ _____
- ◯ _____
- ◯ _____
- ◯ _____

Friday

- ◯ _____
- ◯ _____
- ◯ _____
- ◯ _____
- ◯ _____
- ◯ _____
- ◯ _____
- ◯ _____
- ◯ _____

Saturday

- ◯ _____
- ◯ _____
- ◯ _____
- ◯ _____
- ◯ _____
- ◯ _____
- ◯ _____
- ◯ _____
- ◯ _____

TO-DO LIST

Movement Planner

M	
T	
W	
Th	
F	
S	
Su	

Sunday

- ◯ _____
- ◯ _____
- ◯ _____
- ◯ _____
- ◯ _____
- ◯ _____
- ◯ _____
- ◯ _____
- ◯ _____

TO-DO LIST

Monday

_____ / _____ / _____

Top Priorities

1. _____
2. _____
3. _____

TO-DOS

- ○ _____
- ○ _____
- ○ _____
- ○ _____
- ○ _____
- ○ _____
- ○ _____
- ○ _____
- ○ _____
- ○ _____
- ○ _____

NOTES

MEALS

B	
L	
D	
S	

WATER TRACKER

○ ○ ○ ○ ○ ○ ○ ○ ○

TIME BLOCKING

:	
:	
:	
:	
:	
:	
:	
:	
:	
:	
:	
:	
:	
:	
:	
:	
:	
:	
:	
:	
:	

Tuesday

_____ / _____ / _____

Top Priorities

1. _____

2. _____

3. _____

TO-DOS

- ○ _____
- ○ _____
- ○ _____
- ○ _____
- ○ _____
- ○ _____
- ○ _____
- ○ _____
- ○ _____
- ○ _____
- ○ _____

NOTES

MEALS

B	
L	
D	
S	

WATER TRACKER

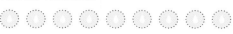

TIME BLOCKING

:	
:	
:	
:	
:	
:	
:	
:	
:	
:	
:	
:	
:	
:	
:	
:	
:	
:	
:	
:	

Wednesday

_____ / _____ / _____

Top Priorities

1. _____
2. _____
3. _____

TO-DOS

- ○ _____
- ○ _____
- ○ _____
- ○ _____
- ○ _____
- ○ _____
- ○ _____
- ○ _____
- ○ _____
- ○ _____
- ○ _____

NOTES

MEALS

B	
L	
D	
S	

WATER TRACKER

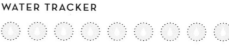

TIME BLOCKING

:	
:	
:	
:	
:	
:	
:	
:	
:	
:	
:	
:	
:	
:	
:	
:	
:	
:	
:	
:	

Thursday

_____ / _____ / _____

Top Priorities

1 _____

2 _____

3 _____

TO-DOS

- ○ _____
- ○ _____
- ○ _____
- ○ _____
- ○ _____
- ○ _____
- ○ _____
- ○ _____
- ○ _____
- ○ _____
- ○ _____

NOTES

MEALS

B	
L	
D	
S	

WATER TRACKER

TIME BLOCKING

:	
:	
:	
:	
:	
:	
:	
:	
:	
:	
:	
:	
:	
:	
:	
:	
:	
:	
:	
:	

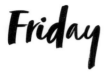

Friday

_____ / _____ / _____

Top Priorities

1. _____
2. _____
3. _____

TO-DOS

- ○ _____
- ○ _____
- ○ _____
- ○ _____
- ○ _____
- ○ _____
- ○ _____
- ○ _____
- ○ _____
- ○ _____

NOTES

MEALS

B	
L	
D	
S	

WATER TRACKER

TIME BLOCKING

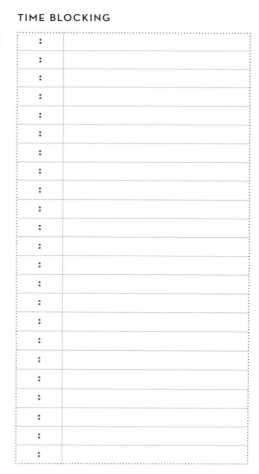

Saturday & Sunday

Top Priorities

1. _____
2. _____
3. _____

MEALS

B	
L	
D	
S	

WATER TRACKER

◉ ◉ ◉ ◉ ◉ ◉ ◉ ◉ ◉

TO-DOS

- ○ _____
- ○ _____
- ○ _____
- ○ _____
- ○ _____
- ○ _____
- ○ _____
- ○ _____
- ○ _____
- ○ _____
- ○ _____

TIME BLOCKING

:	
:	
:	
:	
:	
:	
:	
:	
:	
:	
:	
:	
:	
:	
:	
:	
:	
:	
:	

NOTES

WEEKLY REFLECTION

How do you feel about what you accomplished in the last seven days? What went well?

What do you believe to be the obstacles you faced in accomplishing the goals you set last week?

What would a "win" look like for this coming week?

What steps do you need to take to make your "win" a reality?

Intentional Spending

THE TWENTY-FOUR-HOUR RULE

Intention. This is a word I have been using a lot. Intentionally slowing down. Eating with intention. Moving with intention. Intentional spending is another one to add to the list.

If financial security is a goal of yours, then you have to practice spending with intention. Even the wealthiest of people have a money plan. This means implementing rules to help you stay on track.

One tool I use to foster intentional spending is the twenty-four-hour rule.

Online shopping has been both a blessing and a curse. Targeted ads, social media markets, 50-percent-off emails. We are constantly being bombarded by social media and advertisements telling us: YOU NEED THIS! BUY IT NOW! Our economy thrives on continuous consumption, and I don't foresee that changing anytime soon. But you will never save any money if you recklessly online shop.

When you find yourself accidentally on your favorite department store's website, aimlessly adding things to your cart, try this: Close the browser and wait 24 hours before you buy. One of two things will happen. You will discover that the purchase is warranted, and maybe by waiting you'll end up with a coupon in your inbox to save you some money. But I'm betting in most cases, you will realize that you don't actually need—or even want—what's in your cart and you'll delete it, saving yourself some hard-earned money in the process. Either way, the 24-hour rule will help quell that impulsive, in-need-of-instant-gratification child that lives deep within all of us. If you do that enough times, you'll develop a healthy habit (and you know I love habits), have disposable income that you can invest, and actually make money rather than spend it.

Practice

Do a no-spend challenge. On Sunday, forecast your needs, plan your meals, and go a full seven days without spending money on unnecessary items. No coffee runs, no target stops, no eating out. Plan, budget, execute. After seven days, if it felt easy, continue on for fourteen days or maybe even an entire month. Pay attention to your spending impulses and keep tabs on how much money you save!

How can you be more intentional with your spending? I'm sure 40 percent off is an amazing deal, but do you really need another pair of jeans? Unsubscribing from department store emails can help you curb unintentional spending.

_____

_____

_____

_____

_____

What subscription services are you currently using? Write them down.

Netflix, Spotify, Disney+, Apple TV+, Amazon Prime

_____

_____

_____

They add up! Now write down which ones to keep and which you can cancel.

_____

Are there any other things you're buying that you don't really need? Costco has a way of making that fifteen-pound bag of acai chocolate look tantalizing.

_____

_____

_____

GIVING BACK

Once you make a habit of monitoring your finances, spending intentionally, and investing, you'll find yourself with the wonderful opportunity to give back. And even if you don't have the financial resources to give back just yet, you'll have the gift of time—time for yourself and time for others.

It is statistically proven that people who volunteer regularly are healthier both physically and mentally.[14] Whether it's making sandwiches for a local food pantry or helping raise money for your favorite charity, giving back to your community has been associated with the following health benefits:

- lower blood pressure
- increased self-esteem
- less depression
- lower stress levels
- longer life[15]
- greater happiness and satisfaction

There is also evidence that when you give gifts, you secrete "feel good" chemicals in your brain similar to those that are released during exercise. So not only do you create a stronger community by giving back, but you also create a stronger you! Seems like a no-brainer, in my opinion. How can you give back?

What nonprofit organizations are you passionate about? Research
their volunteer opportunities.

_____

_____

_____

_____

_____

How much time can you realistically dedicate to volunteering at an
organization? How can you rearrange your schedule to make time for
more volunteering?

_____

_____

_____

_____

Name one way you can help someone this week. Put it on your Week-
at-a-Glance and make it happen.

_____

_____

_____

_____

Week-at-a-Glance

TO-DO LIST

Monday

- ◯ _____
- ◯ _____
- ◯ _____
- ◯ _____
- ◯ _____
- ◯ _____
- ◯ _____
- ◯ _____
- ◯ _____

Tuesday

- ◯ _____
- ◯ _____
- ◯ _____
- ◯ _____
- ◯ _____
- ◯ _____
- ◯ _____
- ◯ _____
- ◯ _____

Wednesday

- ◯ _____
- ◯ _____
- ◯ _____
- ◯ _____
- ◯ _____
- ◯ _____
- ◯ _____
- ◯ _____
- ◯ _____

Habit Tracker

HABIT	M	T	W	Th	F	S	Su

What's for Dinner?

M	
T	
W	
Th	
F	
S	
Su	

Thursday

- ◯ _____
- ◯ _____
- ◯ _____
- ◯ _____
- ◯ _____
- ◯ _____
- ◯ _____
- ◯ _____
- ◯ _____

Friday

- ◯ _____
- ◯ _____
- ◯ _____
- ◯ _____
- ◯ _____
- ◯ _____
- ◯ _____
- ◯ _____
- ◯ _____

Saturday

- ◯ _____
- ◯ _____
- ◯ _____
- ◯ _____
- ◯ _____
- ◯ _____
- ◯ _____
- ◯ _____
- ◯ _____

TO-DO LIST

Movement Planner

M	
T	
W	
Th	
F	
S	
Su	

Sunday

- ◯ _____
- ◯ _____
- ◯ _____
- ◯ _____
- ◯ _____
- ◯ _____
- ◯ _____
- ◯ _____
- ◯ _____

TO-DO LIST

Monday

_____ / _____ / _____

Top Priorities

1. _____
2. _____
3. _____

TO-DOS

- ○ _____
- ○ _____
- ○ _____
- ○ _____
- ○ _____
- ○ _____
- ○ _____
- ○ _____
- ○ _____
- ○ _____
- ○ _____

NOTES

MEALS

B	
L	
D	
S	

WATER TRACKER

○ ○ ○ ○ ○ ○ ○ ○ ○

TIME BLOCKING

:	
:	
:	
:	
:	
:	
:	
:	
:	
:	
:	
:	
:	
:	
:	
:	
:	
:	
:	
:	
:	
:	

_____ / ___ / ___

Tuesday

Top Priorities

1. _____
2. _____
3. _____

TO-DOS

- ○ _____
- ○ _____
- ○ _____
- ○ _____
- ○ _____
- ○ _____
- ○ _____
- ○ _____
- ○ _____
- ○ _____

NOTES

MEALS

B	
L	
D	
S	

WATER TRACKER

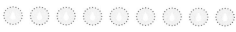

TIME BLOCKING

:	
:	
:	
:	
:	
:	
:	
:	
:	
:	
:	
:	
:	
:	
:	
:	
:	
:	
:	
:	

Wednesday

_____ / _____ / _____

Top Priorities

1. _____
2. _____
3. _____

TO-DOS

- ○ _____
- ○ _____
- ○ _____
- ○ _____
- ○ _____
- ○ _____
- ○ _____
- ○ _____
- ○ _____
- ○ _____
- ○ _____

NOTES

MEALS

B	
L	
D	
S	

WATER TRACKER

○ ○ ○ ○ ○ ○ ○ ○ ○

TIME BLOCKING

:	
:	
:	
:	
:	
:	
:	
:	
:	
:	
:	
:	
:	
:	
:	
:	
:	
:	
:	
:	
:	

_____ / _____ / _____

Thursday

Top Priorities

1. _____
2. _____
3. _____

TO-DOS

- ○ _____
- ○ _____
- ○ _____
- ○ _____
- ○ _____
- ○ _____
- ○ _____
- ○ _____
- ○ _____
- ○ _____
- ○ _____

NOTES

MEALS

B	
L	
D	
S	

WATER TRACKER

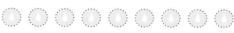

TIME BLOCKING

:	
:	
:	
:	
:	
:	
:	
:	
:	
:	
:	
:	
:	
:	
:	
:	
:	
:	
:	

Friday

_____ / _____ / _____

Top Priorities

1. _____
2. _____
3. _____

TO-DOS

- ○ _____
- ○ _____
- ○ _____
- ○ _____
- ○ _____
- ○ _____
- ○ _____
- ○ _____
- ○ _____
- ○ _____
- ○ _____

NOTES

MEALS

B	
L	
D	
S	

WATER TRACKER

○ ○ ○ ○ ○ ○ ○ ○ ○

TIME BLOCKING

:	
:	
:	
:	
:	
:	
:	
:	
:	
:	
:	
:	
:	
:	
:	
:	
:	
:	
:	
:	
:	

_____ / _____ / _____

Saturday/Sunday

Top Priorities

1. _____
2. _____
3. _____

TO-DOS

- ○ _____
- ○ _____
- ○ _____
- ○ _____
- ○ _____
- ○ _____
- ○ _____
- ○ _____
- ○ _____
- ○ _____
- ○ _____

NOTES

MEALS

B	
L	
D	
S	

WATER TRACKER

○ ○ ○ ○ ○ ○ ○ ○ ○

TIME BLOCKING

:	
:	
:	
:	
:	
:	
:	
:	
:	
:	
:	
:	
:	
:	
:	
:	
:	
:	
:	
:	

WEEKLY REFLECTION

How do you feel about what you accomplished in the last seven days? What went well?

What do you believe to be the obstacles you faced in accomplishing the goals you set last week?

What would a "win" look like for this coming week?

What steps do you need to take to make your "win" a reality?

"To get the results you want, you don't have to be extreme, just consistent."

– UNKNOWN

CONCLUSION

Tying It All Together

Over the past twelve weeks, you have been creating habits and new routines that will give you a strong foundation to improve your physical and mental health, get your finances on track, and connect with your community. If you continue to integrate these into your daily life, you will see an improvement in your overall well-being, which will benefit everyone around you. I'm confident it will happen to you because it happened to me!

I propose using the the prompts on the opposite page to end the twelve-week sessions with a final reflection.

As I said at the beginning, balance is bullshit. Life is complicated and busy and no one can do everything all the time. So if you lose a little momentum or neglect one aspect of the four pillars, don't beat yourself up about it. Instead, pause for a moment, fill in your Week-at-a-Glance and Daily Plan, and continue to move forward. You don't need to achieve perfection—you just need to work toward it to see real improvement and change. You can do it!

What habits have you created that you want to maintain going forward?

_____

_____

_____

_____

_____

_____

_____

_____

What do you need to help you stick to those habits?

_____

_____

_____

_____

_____

_____

_____

_____

RESOURCES

THIRTY DAYS OF JOURNAL PROMPTS

It's always fun to dream about the unimaginable. These prompts are meant to be thought provoking, not necessarily actionable. I believe in the power of manifestation—if you can't think outside the box, you'll forever be trapped in a world less colorful.

1. What habit have I developed that I like? Do I have any habits that I should break? Make a plan to start or stop a habit right now.

2. How can I include fitness and movement in my lifestyle?

3. What is one habit I'd like to start?

4. Something I'd love to do more of in my daily life is . . . How can I make that happen?

5. How do I want to feel when I wake up in the mornings?

6. Plan a week of healthy meals.

7. What is one thing I've really wanted to do? What is stopping me?

8. Plan the week ahead! List three priorities that I want to complete.

9. What makes me feel the most confident?

10. What is my dream career? Write down three things I can do to get closer to that career and implement them.

11. Am I stressed? What is causing it? Write down two ways I might relieve it.

12. Identify and list three things I am grateful for.

13. I feel happy when . . .

14. Think of a song that brings good memories. Write down the name of the song and the memory. Hum that song when I need a pick-me-up.

15. Go completely phone-free for the day. List three things I can do instead of scrolling.

16. If I could live anywhere in the world, where would it be and why? Write down ways I can achieve that.

17. What is one fear I would like to overcome? How can I make that happen?

18. What seems to be missing from my life and what are some potential ways I could get it?

19. Try something new. What is that something? Commit to trying it by a certain date.

20. How could I change one relationship in my life for the better?

21. Make a list of things I have that I don't need any more. What local charities would benefit if I donated them? Make it happen.

22. Am I holding a grudge? Write it down. Now let it go.

23. Write down something good that happened over the weekend. Why did it make me happy?

24. Think of a bucket list travel location. How much would it cost to go there. Set a financial plan to make it happen!

25. Think of the financial goals I have set. Have I moved closer to achieving any of them? What will it mean if I achieve them?

26. What does financial empowerment mean to me?

27. Create a happy list. Write out a list of places or activities that lift my mood.

28. What is my happiest childhood memory?

29. Scan the room. Make note of five things close to me that I am grateful for.

30. What is my favorite smell? Why?

ADDITIONAL MATERIALS

Additional materials and printouts can be found at the following link: **www.liftlikeamother.com/bibresources**

BOOKS TO INCLUDE ON YOUR JOURNEY

Books play a big role in my life. You can always find one in my purse, a habit that I'm happily passing down to my daughter Makayla.

If daily reading is a habit you want to develop, I suggest starting with *The Daily Stoic* by Ryan Holiday. Reading one page each night is sustainable and does not require a lot of time. Eventually, you'll crave more pages and will have a desirable book stack by your bed.

Here are just a few that I have read recently that have impacted my life:

- *Atomic Habits* by James Clear
- *Fit for Success: Lessons on Achievement and Leading Your Best Life* by Nick Shaw
- *How to Be an Antiracist* by Ibram X. Kendi
- *Quit Like a Woman: The Radical Choice to Not Drink in a Culture Obsessed with Alcohol* by Holly Whitaker
- *The 4-Hour Work Week* by Tim Ferriss
- *The Four Agreements* by Don Miguel Ruiz
- *The Psychology of Money* by Morgan Housel
- *Thick and Other Essays* by Tressie McMillan Cottom
- *Untamed* by Glennon Doyle

HEALTHY SHOPPING LIST

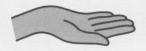

One Handful: CARBOHYDRATES

MACRO: 20–30g

FOOD SCALE EQUIVALENT: ½ – ⅔ cup (100–130g) cooked grains, 1 medium fruit

STARCHY TUBERS
Potatoes (all colors)
Sweet potatoes (all colors)
Taro
Yuca

DAIRY
Plain Kefir
Plain yogurt (not Greek)

WHOLE GRAINS
Brown and wild rice
Barley
Buckwheat
Oats
Quinoa
Wheat berries
Whole or sprouted grain flour foods (breads, bagels, English muffins, pastas, wraps)
Steel-cut or old-fashioned oats
Corn

BEANS & LEGUMES
Beans
Lentils
Peas

FRUITS
Fresh fruit
Frozen fruit
Unsweetened dried fruit

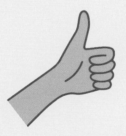

One Thumb: FATS

MACRO: 7–12g

FOOD SCALE EQUIVALENT: 1 tbsp (14g) oils, nuts, seeds, butter, cheese, etc.

NUTS & SEEDS
Almonds
Walnuts
Flax seeds
Sunflower seeds
Chia seeds

OILS & BUTTERS
Extra-virgin olive oil
Nut butters
Coconut oil

OTHER
Avocados
Olives
Eggs
Salmon

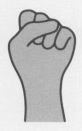

One Fist: VEGETABLES

MACRO: **N/A**

FOOD SCALE EQUIVALENT: **1 cup, non-starchy vegatables**

RED & PINK
Beets
Red cabbage
Red onions
Red leaf lettuce &
    radicchio
Red peppers
Tomatoes
Rhubarb
Raspberries
Salmonberries
Cranberries
Lingonberries
Cherries
Pomegranates
Red grapefruit
Red grapes
Red apples
Strawberries
Watermelon

PURPLE & BLUE
Eggplant
Purple carrots
Purple peppers
Purple cauliflower
Purple asparagus
Purple cabbage
Purple kale
Black cherries
Black currants (fresh)
Black grapes
Black & purple plums
Blueberries
Blackberries

ORANGE & YELLOW
Winte squash varieties
Yellow zucchini &
    summer squash
Pumpkin
Orange & yellow
    peppers
Orange cauliflower
Yellow-orange beets
Apricots, peaches,
    nectarines
Cantaloupe
Mangoes
Oranges
Papayas
Pineapple
Bananas

WHITE
Bean sprouts
Cauliflower
Celery
Daikon radish
Fennel/anise
Garlic
Jicama
Mushrooms
Onions
Leeks
Shallots
Iceberg lettuce
White carrots

GREEN
Broccoli, broccolini
Brussels sprouts
Fresh parsley
Fresh basil
Green beans
Snap peas
Kale
Okra
Spinach
Collard greens
Swiss chard
Arugula
Zucchini
Cucumber
Romaine lettuce
Asparagus
Cabbage
Kiwis

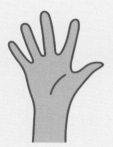

PROTEINS: *One Palm*

MACRO: 20-30g

FOOD SCALE EQUIVALENT: **3-4 oz (85-115g) cooked meat/tofu, 1 cup Greek yogurt**

ANIMAL-BASED
Beef, bison, buffalo
Lean cuts of pork and
    boar
Lamb
Goat
Elk
Venison
Moose
Caribou
Chicken
Turkey
Duck
Pigeon
Fish
Shrimp
Squid
Octopus
Lobster
Crayfish
Clams
Mussels
Scallops
Snails
Eggs and egg whites
Cottage cheese
Strained Greek yogurt

PLANT-BASED
Beans
Lentils
Legumes
Tempeh
Tofu
Edamame
Seitan

SUPPLEMENTS
Protein powder such
    as whey, casein,
    egg, bone broth/
    collagen
Plant-based blends
    (e.g., pea protein,
    rice protein, hemp
    protein)

BAKED LEMON-BUTTER CHICKEN

This is a great recipe to make on a busy weeknight because it's easy, nutritious, and delicious, and the leftovers are amazing.

3 boneless chicken breasts

$\frac{1}{2}$ teaspoon salt plus more for the chicken

1 lemon, zested and juiced

3 tablespoons ghee or butter

$\frac{1}{4}$ cup coconut cream

$\frac{1}{2}$ teaspoon garlic powder

2 tablespoons chopped fresh rosemary

Steamed white rice and green veggies, for serving

Preheat the oven to 375°F.

Place the chicken breasts in a 13-by-9-inch baking pan and sprinkle lightly with salt on both sides. Set the pan aside.

In a medium saucepan, combine the lemon zest and juice, ghee, coconut cream, garlic powder, salt, and rosemary and cook over medium heat, stirring, until the ghee is melted and smooth.

Pour the mixture over the chicken and bake for 40 to 45 minutes, or until the chicken reaches an internal temperature of 165°F.

Serve over steamed white rice with some green veggies and you'll have yourself a tasty, reliable meal that everyone will like (except maybe the really picky ones).

SOURCES

1   Katherine R. Arlinghaus and Craig A. Johnston, "The Importance
    of Creating Habits and Routine, *American Journal of Lifestyle
    Medicine* 13, no. 2 (Mar–Apr 2019): 142–44.

2   Benjamin Gardner, Phillippa Lally, Jane Wardle, "Making Health
    Habitual: The Psychology of 'Habit-Formation' and General
    Practice," *British Journal of General Practice* 62, no. 605 (Dec
    2012): 664–66.

3   Laila AlDabal and Ahmed S. BaHammam, "Betabolic, Endocrine,
    and Innume Consequences of Sleep Deprivation," *The Open
    Respiratory Medicine Journal* 5 (2011): 31–43, https://www.ncbi.nlm.
    nih.gov/pmc/articles/PMC3132857.

4   Ji-Yeong Seo, "The effects of aromatherapy on stress and stress
    responses in adolescents," *Journal of Korean Academy of Nursing*
    39, no. 3 (Jun 2009): 357–365, https://pubmed.ncbi.nlm.nih.
    gov/19571632/.

5   S. Folkard, "Diurnal variation in logical reasoning," *British Journal of
    Psychology* 66, no. 1 (Feb 1975): 1–8, https://pubmed.ncbi.nlm.nih.
    gov/1131476/.

6   Kory Taylor and Elizabeth B. Jones, "Adult Dehydration," *Stat Pearls*
    (Treasure Island, FL: StatPearls Publishing, 2021), https://www.ncbi.
    nlm.nih.gov/books/NBK555956/.

7   American Osteopathic Association, "Group exercise improves
    quality of Life, reduces stress far more than individual work outs,"
    Science Daily, 30 October 2017, https://www.sciencedaily.com/
    releases/2017/10/171030092917.htm.

8   Randy A. Sansone and Lori A. Sansone, "Gratitude and Well Being:
    The Benefits of Appreciation," *Psychiatry* 7, no. 11 (Nov 2010): 18–22,
    https://www.ncbi.nlm.nih.gov/pmc/articles/PMC3010965/; Glenn R.
    Fox, Jonas Kaplan, Hanna Damasio, and Antonio Damasio, "Neural
    Correlates of Gratittude," *Frontiers in Psychology* 6 (2015), https://
    www.frontiersin.org/articles/10.3389/fpsyg.2015.01491/full.

9   Neil Schneiderman, Gail Ironson, and Scott D. Siegel, "Stress and Health: Psychological, Behavioral, and Biological Determinants," *Annual Review of Clinical Psychology* 1 (2005): 607–28, https://www.ncbi.nlm.nih.gov/pmc/articles/PMC2568977/.

10 Jeremy Dean, "Memory Improved 20% by Nature Walk," *PsyBlog*, *January 7*, 2009, https://www.spring.org.uk/2009/01/memory-improved-20-by-nature-walk.php.

11 Jo Barton and Jules Pretty, "What is the best dose of nature and green exercise for improving mental health? A multi-study analysis," *Environmental Science Technology* 44, no. 10 (May 15, 2010): 3947–55, doi: 10.1021/es903183r.

12 Laura Peterson, "Decrease stress by using your breath," Mayo Clinic, March 23, 2017, https://www.mayoclinic.org/healthy-lifestyle/stress-management/in-depth/decrease-stress-by-using-your-breath/art-20267197?pg=2.

13 Daryl B. O'Connor, Sarah Walker, Hilde Hendrickx, Duncan Talbot, and Alexandre Schaefer, "Stress-related thinking predicts the cortisol awakening response and somatic symptoms in healthy adults," *Psychoneuroendocrinology* 38, no. 3 (Mar 2013): 438–46, doi: 10.1016/j.psyneuen.2012.07.004.

14 Ricky N. Lawton, Julian Gramatki, Will Watt, and Daniel Fujiwara, "Does Volunteering Make Us Happier, or Are Happier People More Likely to Volunteer? Addressing the Problem of Reverse Causality When Estimating the Wellbeing Impacts of Volunteering," *Journal of Happiness Studies* 22 (2021): 599–624, doi: 10.1016/j.psyneuen.2012.07.004.

15 University of Michigan, "People who give, live longer: U-M study shows," News release, November 12, 2002, https://www.eurekalert.org/news-releases/887795.

Acknowledgments

As I type this, my eldest daughter is doing a puzzle by the fireplace, my other three children are watching TV, and my husband is cooking lunch for our ever-growing family. I would be nothing without these people, and I feel thankful and blessed every day for the life I live.

This project has been a year in the making, and Angela and the whole Collective Book Studio team are the anchor to my raft. My deepest gratitude to everyone involved, both big and small. It truly takes a village.

And finally, to my mother. You already know the deal. I love you more than life itself.

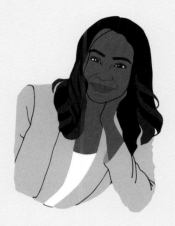

About the Author

Alicia McKenzie, a.k.a. @LiftLikeAMother, is the founder and operator of McKenzie Enterprise LLC, where she has created a premier digital coaching service that focuses on women's holistic health and wellness. In addition, she launched Amplify Health and Wellness Inc., a charitable foundation platform dedicated to empowering the underserved and underrepresented communities by creating health and wellness opportunities that are accessible to all. Its vision is to end the healthy lifestyle and representation poverty gap. She believes that we must work together to create positive and representative healthy role models that can lift up the underserved.

Alicia is a former USA Weightlifting and CrossFit athlete with over a decade in the fitness industry. She has owned and operated CrossFit gyms, is a certified personal trainer, a small business real estate portfolio owner, and most importantly, a mother of five. She has lived the reality of juggling being a business owner, a wife, a mother, and a biracial woman. Contact Alicia at www.liftlikeamother.com.

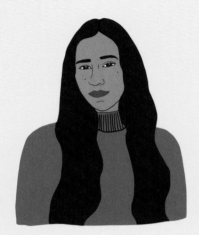

About the Illustrator

Regina Shklovsky is an illustrator and graphic designer based in Sonoma County, California. She illustrated the children's books *Little Loon Finds His Voice* and *Fun in the Mud*, which won a 2019 Moonbeam award and a 2018 Nautilus award, as well as *Embrace the Work, Love Your Career*. Her work is rooted in traditional drawing and painting, mixed with vector graphics.

Library of Congress Cataloging-in-Publication Data available.

ISBN: 978-1-951412-30-2
LCCN: 2021902200

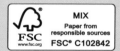

Printed using Forest Stewardship Council certified stock from
sustainably managed forests.

Manufactured in China.

Cover design by David Miles.
Interior design and typesetting by AJ Hansen.
Illustrations by Regina Shklovsky.

10 9 8 7 6 5 4 3 2 1

The Collective Book Studio®
Oakland, California
www.thecollectivebook.studio